AF524871

Management of Pancreatic Neuroendocrine Tumors

Joseph R. Pisegna
Editor

Management of Pancreatic Neuroendocrine Tumors

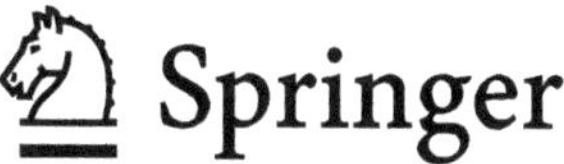

Springer

Editor
Joseph R. Pisegna
David Geffen School of Medicine at UCLA
VA Greater Los Angeles Healthcare System
Los Angeles, CA, USA

ISBN 978-1-4939-1797-6 ISBN 978-1-4939-1798-3 (eBook)
DOI 10.1007/978-1-4939-1798-3
Springer New York Heidelberg Dordrecht London

Library of Congress Control Number: 2014951683

Printed on acid-free paper

Springer is part of Springer Science+Business Media (www.springer.com)

Preface

Neuroendocrine tumors (NETs) are becoming increasingly recognized by both healthcare professionals and patients as being more common than previously recognized. This increased awareness has resulted from increased educational efforts on the part of several societies and patient-supported, nonprofit organizations. We owe much thanks to these educational efforts from dedicated health professionals, patients, and advocates. An increase in federal funding and research support from several nonprofit groups such as Caring for Carcinoid Foundation, the North American Neuroendocrine Tumor Society, and the European Neuroendocrine Tumor Society have positively impacted the field of research. Several pharmaceutical companies, including Novartis, Pfizer, and Ipsen Pharmaceuticals Inc., have provided clinical research funding for new drugs to treat neuroendocrine tumors. As a result of these combined efforts and as reflected in this book, new imaging techniques such as the DOTATATE-Gallium 68 and FDG-PET have improved our ability to detect small, previously unrecognized NETs. We have refined our endoscopic imaging techniques to permit extirpation by endoscopic mucosal resection of small intraluminal NETs such as gastric and rectal carcinoids. The pathology of NETs has been refined which impacts the staging of disease through using molecular markers. We now have a greater understanding of the genetics of NETs, an area which will likely expand in the future. With these improved imaging and histopathological techniques, our surgical colleagues have a greater awareness of tumor staging preceding a planned resection procedure. A greater understanding of the receptor and signaling pathways of NETs has yielded directed chemotherapy and radiopharmaceuticals to treat regional or distant metastases. This book includes 12 chapters that cover these important clinical areas of research and development and has been written by experts in their respective fields. It is my hope that this will be the start of increased awareness for junior investigators and seasoned clinicians to stimulate improvements in research design and therapies which will ultimately translate to improved clinical outcomes for patients with NETs.

Los Angeles, CA, USA — Joseph R. Pisegna, M.D.

Contents

1 **Pathology of Pancreatic Neuroendocrine Tumors** 1
Nils Lambrecht

2 **Inherited and Somatic Genetics of Pancreatic Neuroendocrine Tumors** 9
Lauren Fishbein and Katherine L. Nathanson

3 **Laboratory Assessment of NETs** 33
Christos Toumpanakis

4 **Zollinger–Ellison Syndrome: Diagnosis and Management** 41
Maneesh H. Singh and David C. Metz

5 **Clinical Manifestations of Multiple Endocrine Neoplasia, Type 1** 63
Susan Yuditskaya and Monica C. Skarulis

6 **Gastric Carcinoids: Classification and Diagnosis** 83
Kali Zhou and Wendy Ho

7 **Endoscopic Approaches for Diagnosis of Pancreatic Neuroendocrine Tumors** 95
Tarun Rustagi and James J. Farrell

8 **Endoscopic Approaches to Treatment of Pancreatic Neuroendocrine Neoplasms** 111
Amit Raina and Vinay Chandrasekhara

9 **Surgical Approaches to Pancreatic Neuroendocrine Tumors** 117
James X. Wu and F. Charles Brunicardi

10 **Radiotherapy and Radiopharmaceuticals for the Treatment of Pancreatic Neuroendocrine Tumors** 127
Lowell B. Anthony and Partha Sinha

11 Nuclear Medicine Approaches to Treatment of Neuroendocrine Tumors 135
Ken Herrmann, Rudolf A. Werner, Christina Blümel, and Martin S. Allen-Auerbach

12 Novel Targets for Future Medical Treatments 145
Sandy T. Liu, Andrew E. Hendifar, and Edward M. Wolin

Index 163

Contributors

Martin S. Allen-Auerbach Department of Molecular and Medical Pharmacology, UCLA Medical Center, Los Angeles, CA, USA

Lowell B. Anthony Division of Medical Oncology, Markey Cancer Center, University of Kentucky, Lexington, KY, USA

Christina Blümel Department of Nuclear Medicine, Universitätsklinikum Würzburg, Würzburg, Germany

F. Charles Brunicardi Ronald Reagan UCLA Medical Center, Los Angeles, CA, USA

UCLA Medical Center, Santa Monica, CA, USA

Vinay Chandrasekhara Gastroenterology Division, University of Pennsylvania Health System, Philadelphia, PA, USA

James J. Farrell Yale Center for Pancreatic Disease, Yale University School of Medicine, New Haven, CT, USA

Section of Digestive Diseases, Yale University School of Medicine, New Haven, CT, USA

Lauren Fishbein Division of Endocrinology, Diabetes and Metabolism, Department of Medicine, Perelman School of Medicine at the University of Pennsylvania, Philadelphia, PA, USA

Andrew E. Hendifar Department of Gastrointestinal Oncology, Samuel Oschin Cancer Center, Cedars-Sinai Medical Center, Los Angeles, CA, USA

Ken Herrmann Department of Nuclear Medicine, Universitätsklinikum Würzburg, Würzburg, Germany

Wendy Ho Department of Medicine, Division of Digestive Diseases, UCLA, Los Angeles, CA, USA

Nils Lambrecht Department of Pathology and Laboratory Medicine Service, Long Beach VA Medical, Long Beach, CA, USA

Sandy T. Liu Department of Medicine, Cedars-Sinai Medical Center, Los Angeles, CA, USA

David C. Metz Department of Internal Medicine, Perelman School of Medicine at the University of Pennsylvania, Philadelphia, PA, USA

Division of Gastroenterology, Perelman School of Medicine at the University of Pennsylvania, Philadelphia, PA, USA

Katherine L. Nathanson Division of Translational Medicine and Human Genetics, Department of Medicine, Perelman School of Medicine at the University of Pennsylvania, Philadelphia, PA, USA

Amit Raina Gastroenterology Division, East Carolina University, Greenville, NC, USA

Tarun Rustagi Yale Center for Pancreatic Disease, Yale University School of Medicine, New Haven, CT, USA

Section of Digestive Diseases, Yale University School of Medicine, New Haven, CT, USA

Maneesh H. Singh Department of Internal Medicine, Division of Gastroenterology, University of California, San Francisco, San Francisco, CA, USA

Partha Sinha Division of Nuclear Medicine, Department of Radiology, University of Kentucky, Lexington, KY, USA

Monica C. Skarulis Diabetes, Endocrine, and Obesity Branch, National Institute of Diabetes, Digestive and Kidney Diseases, National Institutes of Health, Bethesda, MD, USA

Christos Toumpanakis Centre for Gastroenterology, Neuroendocrine Tumour Unit, Royal Free Hospital, London, UK

Rudolf A. Werner Department of Nuclear Medicine, Universitätsklinikum Würzburg, Würzburg, Germany

Edward M. Wolin Carcinoid and Neuroendocrine Tumor Program Medical Oncology, Samuel Oschin Cancer Center, Cedars-Sinai Medical Center, Los Angeles, CA, USA

James X. Wu Ronald Reagan UCLA Medical Center, Los Angeles, CA, USA

Susan Yuditskaya Diabetes, Endocrine, and Obesity Branch, National Institute of Diabetes, Digestive and Kidney Diseases, National Institutes of Health, Bethesda, MD, USA

Kali Zhou Department of Medicine, UCLA, Los Angeles, CA, USA

Chapter 1
Pathology of Pancreatic Neuroendocrine Tumors

Nils Lambrecht

1.1 Introduction

Pancreatic neuroendocrine neoplasms have long fascinated clinicians and pathologists, because tumors with similar histopathological appearance can present with distinct clinical syndromes caused by the release of endocrine hormones into the central circulation. In the past, these neoplasms have been classified based on their clinical functional status of hormone secretory or nonsecretory [1]. However, with the availability of long-term patient survival data (SEERS database), it is now unequivocally demonstrated that an accurate estimate of a patient's length of survival is determined by the grade and stage of the tumor and not its functional status. This is reflected in the current grading and staging systems as proposed by the WHO classification of neuroendocrine neoplasms of the pancreas [2], the European Neuroendocrine Tumour Society TNM classification of GEP-NEN (ENETS 2007 [3]), and the US TNM classification tumors (AJCC 2010 [4]). Accordingly, the pathological evaluation of pancreatic neuroendocrine neoplasms is focused on grade and stage, while functional status should only be supplemented if a clinical syndrome is recognized.

1.2 Classification

1.2.1 Nomenclature

The international community has used differing nomenclature to describe pancreatic neuroendocrine neoplasms.

N. Lambrecht (✉)
Department of Pathology and Laboratory Medicine Service,
Long Beach VA Medical, Long Beach, CA, USA
e-mail: Nils.Lambrecht2@va.gov

J.R. Pisegna (ed.), *Management of Pancreatic Neuroendocrine Tumors*,
DOI 10.1007/978-1-4939-1798-3_1

1.2.1.1 Neuroendocrine vs. Endocrine

A series of molecular studies on native pancreatic and gastrointestinal endocrine cells disproved the embryological origin of cells from the neuroectoderm. They are now believed to be derived from the endoderm [5]. Therefore, the term endocrine appears to be biologically correct. However, neoplastic cells do possess histological and molecular features of neural differentiation and the latest 2010 WHO classification adopted the term neuroendocrine once again. In practice, both terms can be used synonymously.

1.2.1.2 Neuroendocrine Tumor vs. Neoplasm

Although the term neoplasm is biologically correct and separates neoplastic lesions from benign non-neoplastic endocrine hyperplasia, the term neuroendocrine tumor has been widely used and is the preferred term for low grade (G1–G2) neuroendocrine neoplasms in the current classification adopted by the current WHO classification (2010) and the TNM staging system (AJCC 2010).

1.2.2 WHO Classification 2010

The current WHO classification has unified the classification of all neuroendocrine neoplasms of the gastrointestinal tract and pancreas, which are now named gastroenteropancreatic neuroendocrine neoplasms (GEP-NEN). They emphasize the notion that all neuroendocrine neoplasms have a malignant potential and should never be regarded as benign. The classification separates low and intermediate grade neuroendocrine tumors (GEP-NET grade 1 and 2, Fig. 1.1) from neuroendocrine carcinomas (GEP-NEC grade 3) and recognizes mixed adenoneuroendocrine carcinomas (Fig. 1.2) as a separate category. In addition, neuroendocrine hyperplasia is now identified as a separate hyperplastic or pre-neoplastic category (Table 1.1).

In order to grade GEP-NENs, the WHO 2010 classification suggests using the current method of grading outlined by the European Neuroendocrine Tumour Society TNM classification of GEP-NEN (ENETS 2007). It is important to note that in order to define a low grade GEP-NET (G1) at a minimum, one has to count less than two mitoses in ten high power fields (400× magnification, hpf) *and* perform a Ki67 immunostain showing less than 3 % of tumor cell nuclei labeled (Fig. 1.1).

1.2.3 TNM Stage: Differences in ENETS 2007 and AJCC 2010 [6]

The European Neuroendocrine Tumour Society TNM classification of GEP-NEN (ENETS 2007) is compatible with the US TNM classification of neuroendocrine tumors of the gastrointestinal tract (AJCC 2010) only for GEP-NETs grades 1 and 2

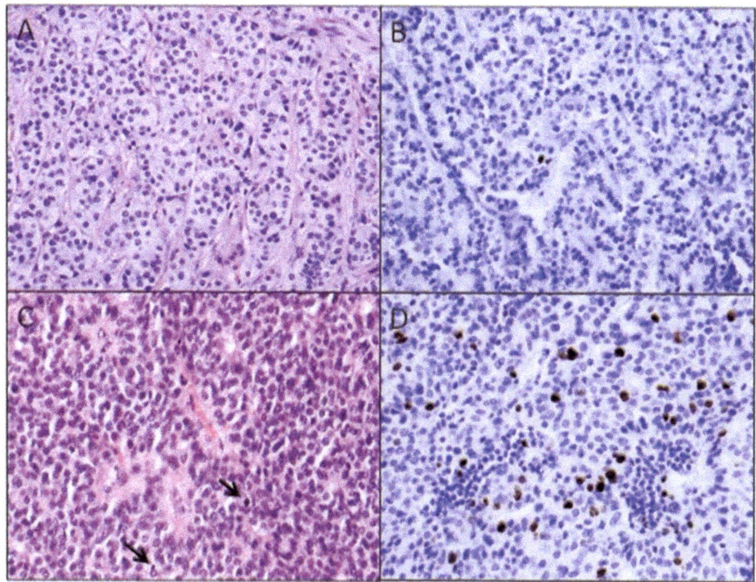

Fig. 1.1 Differences in morphology and Ki67 mitotic index immunolabeling of sections of low grade (G1, panel **a** and **b**) and intermediate grade (G2, panel **c** and **d**) pancreatic neuroendocrine tumors. Panel **c** shows an intermediate grade tumor with higher N:C ratio and increased mitotic rate (*black arrows* highlight mitotic figures). Panel **d** shows that ~5 % of the tumor cells express Ki67 (**a**, **c**) H&E stain 400× magnification; (**b**, **d**) Ki67 immunostain, 400× magnification)

Tumor Grade (WHO 2010)	ENETS 2007
G1-Low grade	<2 mitoses / 10 hpf AND <3% Ki67 index
G2-Intermediate grade	2-20 mitoses / 10 hpf OR 3%-20% Ki67 index
G3-High grade	>20 mitoses / 10 hpf OR >20% Ki67 index

except for pancreatic and appendiceal NETs. It is not compatible for neuroendocrine carcinomas (GEP-NEC, grade 3) of all sites. Table 1.2 lists the two TNM classifications for pancreatic neuroendocrine neoplasms side by side.

1.3 Macroscopic Features (T Stage)

Gross examination of excision specimens should focus on correct determination of the maximal size of the tumor, its local involvement of peripancreatic tissue, and its invasion into major vascular structures (AJCC 2010). The tumor can be well circumscribed or show infiltrative borders. The cut surface is tan-red and homogenous. Tumor necrosis should be mentioned if observed grossly. If invasion into bile duct or duodenum is seen, it should be mentioned in the pathology report to be able to compare European and North American data sets for future outcome studies.

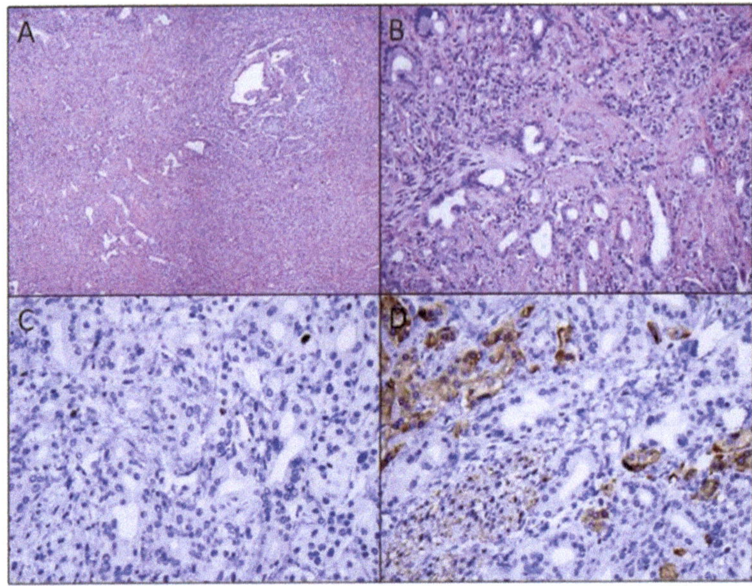

Fig. 1.2 Mixed adenoneuroendocrine carcinoma (MANEC). Panel **a** and **b** show that ~ 50 % of the tumor is comprised of endocrine nests admixed with 50 % exocrine glands with focal perineural invasion. Panel **c** shows low mitotic activity of the tumor. Panel **d** demonstrates that only the endocrine and not the exocrine component expresses synaptophysin (**a**) H&E stain 40× magnification; (**b**) H&E stain 400× magnification; (**c**) Ki67 immunostain, 400× magnification, (**d**) synaptophysin immunostain, 400× magnification)

Table 1.1 Differences in previous and current WHO classifications for gastroenteropancreatic neoplasms

WHO 2000	WHO 2010
Tumor-like lesions (TLL)	Hyperplastic and pre-neoplastic lesions
Well-differentiated endocrine tumor (WDET)	Neuroendocrine tumor grade 1 (GEP-NET)
Well-differentiated endocrine carcinoma (WDEC)	Neuroendocrine tumor grade 2 (GEP-NET)
Poorly differentiated endocrine carcinoma/ small cell carcinoma (PDET)	Neuroendocrine carcinoma grade 3 (GEP-NEC) (large cell or small cell type)
Mixed exocrine endocrine carcinoma (MEEC)	Mixed adenoneuroendocrine carcinoma (MANEC)

Table 1.2 Differences in European and North American tumor staging for gastroenteropancreatic neoplasms

	ENETS TNM 2007	AJCC TNM 2010
T1	Confined to pancreas (<2 cm)	Confined to pancreas (<2 cm)
T2	Confined to pancreas (2–4 cm)	Confined to pancreas (>2 cm)
T3	Confined to pancreas (>4 cm) OR Invasion of duodenum or bile duct	Peripancreatic spread WITHOUT Major vascular invasion
T4	Invasion of adjacent organs OR Major vascular invasion	Major vascular invasion

1.4 Histology (NET vs. NEC, Grade)

Microscopic examination is used to determine the grade of the neuroendocrine neoplasm. Neuroendocrine tumors show classical patterns of neuroendocrine differentiation including organoid (nested), pseudorossetting, trabecular, and solid growth patterns (Fig. 1.3a–d, respectively). They are composed of small uniform cells with round to oval nuclei demonstrating coarsely stippled chromatin ("salt and pepper," Fig. 1.3a insert). The classical term "carcinoid tumor" is still in clinical use but should be qualified with the newer terms of neuroendocrine tumor grade 1 or 2. Large cell neuroendocrine carcinomas show frequently sheet-like solid growth patterns, tumor necrosis, hyperchromatic nuclei, and irregular nuclear contours. Small cell carcinomas lack cytoplasm and demonstrate nuclear molding in addition to tumor necrosis.

In order to determine the grade of the tumor, special emphasize is given to an accurate mitotic count. It is recommended to count 40–50 high power fields (hpf) and calculate the mean of the total number of mitosis in 10 hpf. If the number is less than 2 (G1), the result must be supported by an additional immunohistochemical stain using the proliferative index marker Ki67. Less than 3 % of tumor cells should be positive to qualify the tumor as low grade (G1, Fig. 1.1).

Finally, if a glandular component is seen in more than 30 % of the neuroendocrine carcinoma, the diagnosis of a mixed adenoneuroendocrine carcinoma (MANEC) is

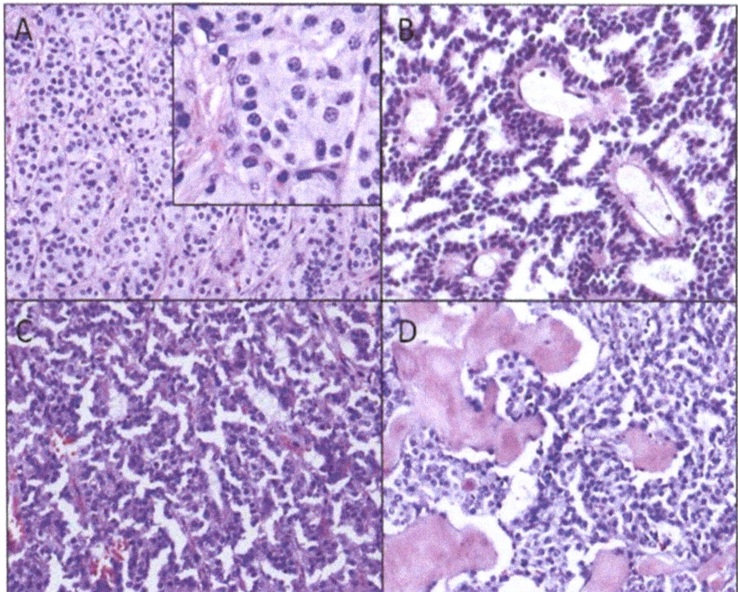

Fig. 1.3 Various growth patterns of neuroendocrine tumors: (**a**) organoid (nested), (**b**) perivascular pseudorosettes, (**c**) trabecular and micropapillary, (**d**) solid with amyloid production (**a**–**c** H&E stain, 400× magnification)

made and grading is performed on the two components separately (Fig. 1.2). If a pancreatic exocrine adenocarcinoma contains less than 30 % of tumor showing neuroendocrine histology and immunostaining, the carcinoma is called adenocarcinoma with focal neuroendocrine differentiation.

1.5 Molecular Marker Expression

A minimal immunohistochemical panel should demonstrate cytoplasmic expression of synaptophysin and chromogranin. Small cell carcinomas show in addition a highly specific perinuclear dot-like staining pattern if an anti-pankeratin (AE1/3) antibody is used.

The presence of somatostatin receptor subtype 2 (SSTR2) on the tumor cells should be determined, since clinically used somatostatin analogues (octreotide, lanreotide) bind with high affinity to somatostatin receptor subtype 2 and with lesser affinity to subtype 3 and 5. The presence of SSTR2 receptors results in higher sensitivity to somatostatin analogue receptor scintigraphy (^{111}In or ^{99}Tc) or PET (^{68}Ga) to correctly detect and stage disease and to estimate effectiveness of treatment by somatostatin analogues.

Finally, rare metastatic tumors to the pancreas from a lung primary can be identified using an anti-TTF1 antibody or from intestinal primaries using an anti-CDX2 antibody. Most primary pancreatic neuroendocrine tumors show expression of PDX-1, which is negative in most neuroendocrine tumors from other sites.

1.6 Molecular Genetics

The overall incidence of pancreatic neuroendocrine tumors worldwide is 1 in 100,000 [7]. Recently, this incidence has been increasing up to 5 in 100,000 most likely due to better detection methods [8]. This is supported by autopsy studies which estimate up to 0.8–3 % of cases showing pancreatic NETs [9, 10]. Most are sporadic, but familial germline mutations exist.

1.6.1 Familial Syndromes

The multiple endocrine neoplasia type 1 gene (MEN1) codes for the protein MENIN, a nuclear transcriptional regulator and tumor suppressor. The gene resides on the long arm of chromosome 11 (11q13). Germline mutations of MEN1 are present in 70–90 % of typical MEN1 families [11].

Another target gene for germline mutations resulting in frequent pancreatic NETs is the von Hippel–Lindau (VHL) gene. This gene resides on the short arm of chromosome 3 (3p25). The VHL protein is found in the nucleus and the cytoplasm and appears to degrade HIF (hypoxia inducible factor). Absence of VHL protein causes overexpression of HIF with production of VEGF and other factors promoting vascular proliferation during tumor development. 15–17 % of patients with VHL germline mutations develop pancreatic PETs and many of these tumors show a more aggressive clinical behavior [12, 13].

Germline mutations in neurofibromatosis type 1 gene (17q11) and tuberous sclerosis genes TSC1 (9q34) and TSC2 (16p13) cause absence of neurofibromin, hamartin, or tuberin, respectively. This causes uncontrolled activation of mTOR and activation of HIF similarly to the absence of the VHL protein. Pancreatic NETs are seen in 6 % of neurofibromatosis type 1 (von Recklinghausen's disease) and less than 5 % of tuberous sclerosis [14].

1.6.2 Sporadic Pancreatic Endocrine Neoplasms

Like in the familial counterparts, loss of heterozygosity (LOH) of chromosome 11q13 was shown in 33–40 % of sporadic pancreatic NETs (33–40 % [15, 16]). This region contains the tumor suppressor gene MENIN (MEN1). Further mutational analysis of the MEN1 gene in cases of absent 11q13 LOH revealed additional heterozygous mutations. This raises the question of haplo-insufficiency of the MEN1 gene to enable tumor suppression [15].

Recently, it has been shown that sporadic pancreatic NETs also show either LOH or other molecular alterations on the short arm of chromosome 3 (3p24–26). Currently, it is not clear if these changes occur as mutations in the VHL gene or promoter region or if other candidate tumor suppressor genes including PPAR, RASSF1A, or others are mutated [12, 13, 17].

References

1. Fendrich V, Waldmann J, Bartsch DK, Langer P. Surgical management of pancreatic endocrine tumors. Nat Rev. 2009;6(7):419–28.
2. Klimstra DS, Arnold R, Capella C, Hruban RH, Klöppel G. Neuroendocrine neoplasms of the pancreas. In: Bosman FT, Carneiro F, Hruban RH, Theise ND, editors. WHO classification of tumours of the digestive system. Lyon: International Agency for Research on Cancer (IARC); 2010. p. 322–26.
3. Rindi G, Kloppel G, Couvelard A, Komminoth P, Korner M, Lopes JM, et al. TNM staging of midgut and hindgut (neuro) endocrine tumors: a consensus proposal including a grading system. Virchows Arch. 2007;451(4):757–62.
4. AJCC Cancer Staging Manual, American Joint Committee on Cancer, 7th. Edition; pp 181–185; pp 241–246; Springer New York Dordrecht Heidelberg London.
5. Oliver-Krasinski JM, Stoffers DA. On the origin of the beta cell. Genes Dev. 2008; 22(15):1998–2021.
6. Kloppel G. Classification and pathology of gastroenteropancreatic neuroendocrine neoplasms. Endocr Relat Cancer. 2011;18 Suppl 1:S1–16.

7. Ehehalt F, Saeger HD, Schmidt CM, Grutzmann R. Neuroendocrine tumors of the pancreas. Oncologist. 2009;14(5):456–67.
8. Haugvik SP, Labori KJ, Edwin B, Mathisen O, Gladhaug IP. Surgical treatment of sporadic pancreatic neuroendocrine tumors: a state of the art review. ScientificWorldJournal. 2012; 2012:357475.
9. Grimelius L, Hultquist GT, Stenkvist B. Cytological differentiation of asymptomatic pancreatic islet cell tumours in autopsy material. Virchows Arch. 1975;365(4):275–88.
10. Kimura W, Kuroda A, Morioka Y. Clinical pathology of endocrine tumors of the pancreas. Analysis of autopsy cases. Dig Dis Sci. 1991;36(7):933–42.
11. Starker LF, Carling T. Molecular genetics of gastroenteropancreatic neuroendocrine tumors. Curr Opin Oncol. 2009;21(1):29–33.
12. Amato E, Barbi S, Malpeli G, Bersani S, Pelosi G, Capelli P, et al. Chromosome 3p alterations in pancreatic endocrine neoplasia. Virchows Arch. 2011;458(1):39–45.
13. Schmitt AM, Schmid S, Rudolph T, Anlauf M, Prinz C, Kloppel G, et al. VHL inactivation is an important pathway for the development of malignant sporadic pancreatic endocrine tumors. Endocr Relat Cancer. 2009;16(4):1219–27.
14. Chen M, Van Ness M, Guo Y, Gregg J. Molecular pathology of pancreatic neuroendocrine tumors. J Gastrointest Oncol. 2012;3(3):182–8.
15. Hessman O, Lindberg D, Einarsson A, Lillhager P, Carling T, Grimelius L, et al. Genetic alterations on 3p, 11q13, and 18q in nonfamilial and MEN 1-associated pancreatic endocrine tumors. Genes Chromosomes Cancer. 1999;26(3):258–64.
16. Wang EH, Ebrahimi SA, Wu AY, Kashefi C, Passaro Jr E, Sawicki MP. Mutation of the MENIN gene in sporadic pancreatic endocrine tumors. Cancer Res. 1998;58(19):4417–20.
17. Chung DC, Smith AP, Louis DN, Graeme-Cook F, Warshaw AL, Arnold A. A novel pancreatic endocrine tumor suppressor gene locus on chromosome 3p with clinical prognostic implications. J Clin Invest. 1997;100(2):404–10.

Chapter 2
Inherited and Somatic Genetics of Pancreatic Neuroendocrine Tumors

Lauren Fishbein and Katherine L. Nathanson

2.1 Introduction

Pancreatic neuroendocrine tumors (PNETs) are tumors derived from endocrine cells of the pancreas found in the islets of Langerhans. PNETs are rare tumors with an incidence in the United States of 3.65 per 100,000 [1]. On autopsy studies, up to 10 % of individuals have PNETs, suggesting many tumors remain undiagnosed [2]. PNETs can occur at any age, with a peak incidence in the fourth to sixth decades of life, and are believed to follow a classic model of tumor progression. The tumors are broadly classified into functional (15 %) and nonfunctional (85 %) PNETs, based on whether they can retain the ability to release one or more hormones such as insulin, gastrin, or glucagon. Nonfunctional PNETs have a worse prognosis, likely due to relative delay in diagnosis, as they are usually discovered at later stages and often are more poorly differentiated [3, 4]. The most common functional tumor, the insulinoma, often is diagnosed while still small and localized because of the severity of symptoms associated with insulin hypersecretion, and thus, the five-year survival rate is quite high at 85–95 %. Seventy percent of patients with the more common nonfunctional tumors present with unresectable disease, often with liver metastases, and the five-year survival rate is only 30–40 % with a median survival of 24 months [1, 5–7]. However, in centers dedicated to neuroendocrine tumor treatment, the five-year survival rate for metastatic disease can be as high as 60 % [8]. For this reason, consensus guidelines from the North American Neuroendocrine Tumor Society

L. Fishbein, M.D., Ph.D. (✉)
Division of Endocrinology, Diabetes and Metabolism, Department of Medicine,
Perelman School of Medicine at the University of Pennsylvania, Philadelphia, PA, USA
e-mail: Lauren.Fishbein@uphs.upenn.edu

K.L. Nathanson, M.D.
Division of Translational Medicine and Human Genetics, Department of Medicine,
Perelman School of Medicine at the University of Pennsylvania, Philadelphia, PA, USA

J.R. Pisegna (ed.), *Management of Pancreatic Neuroendocrine Tumors*,
DOI 10.1007/978-1-4939-1798-3_2

(NANETS) recommend that all patients with metastatic PNETs be treated at specialized centers [9].

The poor prognosis for patients with metastatic or regional disease underscores the urgent need for more effective therapies. As PNETs are relatively rare tumors, the impetus to study their tumor biology has been limited. However, recent technology has allowed for broad-based genetic studies, which have identified novel biomarkers and increased our understanding of tumorigenesis. A thorough understanding of the molecular biology and tumor genetics of PNETs may lead to discovery of novel targets for therapeutic intervention. The goal of this chapter is to summarize the current understanding of inherited and somatic genetics in PNETs.

2.2 Inherited Syndromes Associated with PNETs

Approximately 10–15 % of PNETs are associated with inherited cancer susceptibility syndromes including Multiple Endocrine Neoplasia type 1 (MEN1), von Hippel–Lindau syndrome (vHL), and more rarely Neurofibromatosis type 1 (NF1) and Tuberous Sclerosis Complex (TSC) (Table 2.1).

2.3 MEN1 Syndrome

Multiple Endocrine Neoplasia type 1 (MEN1) is an autosomal dominant cancer susceptibility syndrome, which has an incidence of approximately 0.25 % [10]. In most cases, the syndrome is caused by an inherited germline mutation in the *MEN1* gene. MEN1 is defined by the presence of parathyroid adenomas or hyperplasia, gastroenteropancreatic tumors (GEPNETs), and anterior pituitary adenomas [10]. Hypercalcemia from primary hyperparathyroidism is often the presenting feature of MEN1, and it occurs in almost 100 % of cases by age 50 and often affects all four parathyroid glands. MEN1-associated primary hyperparathyroidism develops at an earlier age than sporadic primary hyperparathyroidism (20–25 years old vs. 55 years old, respectively) [10]. Patients who do not have primary hyperparathyroidism by age 50 have not been found to carry mutations in *MEN1*. Pituitary adenomas occur in up to 60 % of patients with MEN1. Lactotroph adenomas are the most common anterior pituitary tumor observed; somatotroph and somatomammotroph adenomas occur in 5 % of associated pituitary adenomas [11, 12]. Approximately 10 % of MEN1 patients have bronchial or thymic carcinoids and 20–40 % have adrenal cortical tumors. Other non-cancer features include facial angiofibromas, collagenomas, lipomas, and leiomyomas. Of note, both angiofibromas and collagenomas also are observed in TSC. However, patients with MEN1 have fewer angiofibromas, which tend to be non-erythematous and located on the nose rather than nasolabial folds. PNETs are a common feature of MEN1, present in 40–80 % of patients [10, 13]. Mutations in *MEN1* are the most common inherited mutations

Table 2.1 Inherited PNET predisposition genes

Gene	Loci	Protein	Function	Syndrome
MEN1	11q13.1	Menin	Regulates cellular proliferation Role in genomic stability Role in epigenetic regulation	Multiple Endocrine Neoplasia type 1 Hyperparathyroidism GEPNETs Pituitary adenomas Bronchial carcinoids Adrenal adenomas Angiofibromas
VHL	3p25.3	von Hippel–Lindau protein	Negatively regulates HIF by targeting it for ubiquitination and degradation	von Hippel–Lindau Disease Hemangioblastomas of the CNS Endolyphatic sac tumors Epididymal cystadenomas Pheochromocytomas Renal cell carcinomas Pancreatic cysts PNETs
NF1	17q11.2	Neurofibromin	Acts as a GTPase to inactivate Ras to regulate the MAPK pathway	Neurofibromatosis type 1 Cutaneous neurofibromas Plexiform neurofibromas Café-au-lait spots Lisch nodules (benign iris hamartoma) Inguinal or axillary freckling Long bone dysplasia Optic gliomas Rare PNETs
TSC1	9q34	Hamartin	Dimerizes with tuberin to control cellular proliferation through the PI3K/mTOR pathway	Tuberous Sclerosis Complex Facial angiofibromas Ungula fibromas Hypomelanotic macules Renal angiomyolipomas Hamartomas Neurological disorders Rare PNETs
TSC2	16p13.3	Tuberin	Dimerizes with hamartin to control cellular proliferation through the PI3K/mTOR pathway	Tuberous Sclerosis Complex Facial angiofibromas Ungula fibromas Hypomelanotic macules Renal angiomyolipomas Hamartomas Neurological disorders Rare PNETs

leading to increased susceptibility to PNETs. PNETs in MEN1 patients are typically diagnosed at an earlier age (30–50 years old) than in patients with sporadic PNETs, which may represent a screening bias. PNETs associated with MEN1 are often multiple and small (defined as less than 0.5 cm) and most are nonfunctional. Gastrinomas and insulinomas are the most common functional PNETs (40 % and 10 %, respectively) found in MEN1 patients; glucagonomas, VIPomas and somatostatinomas are rare [11, 14]. MEN1 patients with PNETs tend to have a better prognosis than patients with PNETs without MEN1, likely reflecting a screening bias and earlier diagnosis in patients with MEN1. Approximately 10 % of all PNETs and 25 % of gastrinomas (Zollinger–Ellison syndrome) occur in patients with MEN1.

MEN1 demonstrates variable expressivity. Members of the same family, who carry the same mutation, can have diverse clinical manifestations. Identifying individuals with *MEN1* mutations is not only important for the proband's medical management but also for testing family members. Genetic testing is an important medical management tool, and screening and surveillance for the clinical manifestations of disease can be initiated once a mutation is identified. Additionally, having mutational information will allow for preconception genetic counseling and testing, such as preimplantation genetic diagnosis. Finally, identifying individuals in the kindred who do not carry the familial mutation (true negatives) is critical as well, since they do not need lifelong screening for tumors.

2.4 *MEN1* Gene and Mutations

MEN1 is located on chromosome 11q13 and is comprised of ten exons spanning over 7 kb of genomic DNA [15]. The coding region spans 1,830 bp and encodes the protein menin, which is 610 amino acids. Tumors have one germline mutation in *MEN1* with a second hit, often being loss of heterozygosity (LOH), at the other allele. Mutations occur throughout the gene [16, 17]. More than 1,336 different *MEN1* mutations have been reported, both germline (N=1,133) and somatic (N=203) [17]. The 1,133 germline mutations reported in 2008 were found throughout the entire coding region and splice sites. Of the 459 unique mutations, 23 % were nonsense, 41 % frameshift deletions or insertions, 6 % in-frame deletions or insertions, 9 % splice-site mutations, 20 % missense mutations, and 1 % whole or partial gene deletions [17]. Approximately 5–10 % of patients, who meet the clinical diagnostic criteria for MEN1, do not have an identifiable mutation in the coding region of *MEN1* [15–18]. These patients may have mutations in the regulatory regions, such as the promoter, which are not routinely evaluated with clinical genetic testing.

Despite the absence of hotspot mutations in the *MEN1* gene, mutations at nine sites account for 20 % of all germline mutations [17]. Five of these nine mutations are deletions or insertions, one is a novel splice-site acceptor, and three are nonsense mutations. It is hypothesized that the *MEN1* deletion/insertion mutations are caused by replication slippage at areas of repetitive sequence in the gene. There are 24 known polymorphisms in the *MEN1* gene, including two nonsynonymous amino acid changes, which must be differentiated from mutations in clinical genetic testing [17].

2.5 Somatic *MEN1* Mutations

MEN1 is the most common somatically mutated gene in sporadic PNETs, often accompanied by loss of heterozygosity at the second hit. Whole-exome sequencing of ten sporadic PNETs and subsequent targeted sequencing of an additional 58 sporadic PNETs in a validation set found that 44 % had somatic mutations in *MEN1* [19]. These data are consistent with prior work showing that somatic mutations in *MEN1* were found in 30 % of sporadic PNETs, 7 % of insulinomas, 36 % of gastrinomas, 67 % of glucagonomas, and 44 % of VIPomas [20, 21]. As with the known germline mutations, the somatic mutations are scattered throughout the coding sequencing, and 18 % are nonsense mutations, 40 % are frameshift deletions or insertions, 6 % are in-frame deletions or insertions, 7 % are splice-site mutations, and 29 % are missense mutations [17]. Losses of heterozygosity of segments of chromosome 11 (over the *MEN1* locus) have been seen in 38.6 % of nonfunctioning PNETs and 15–20 % of gastrinomas and insulinomas [22, 23]. Most *MEN1* mutations in sporadic PNETs appear to be associated with regions of the gene involved in nuclear localization or protein–protein interactions, and these tumors tend to have abnormally low to absent nuclear staining of menin [21].

2.6 Menin Protein

The *MEN1* gene product, menin, is ubiquitously expressed but functions in a tissue-specific manner, sometimes with opposing functions. Menin is primarily located in the nucleus of nondividing cells and is found in the cytoplasm of dividing cells [24]. Many protein partners have been reported to interact with menin, suggesting a role in various cellular pathways, including the regulation of gene transcription, DNA replication and repair, and signal transduction. Given the wide range of proposed functions and associated protein partners for menin, the discussion below will focus on those pathways and associations most related to neuroendocrine tumorigenesis (Fig. 2.1).

In cell culture, menin represses telomerase activity via interaction with human telomerase reverse transcriptase (hTERT), thereby preventing uncontrolled continued cellular proliferation [25]. Consistent with these data, menin depletion results in immortalization of human fibroblasts [25]. Menin also binds directly to AKT1 to inhibit the PI3K-Akt-mTOR signaling pathway, thereby suppressing proliferation and anti-apoptotic signals [26]. Menin interacts with NF-κB family members to repress the NF-κB-mediated transcriptional activation which is linked to apoptosis and delayed cellular growth [27]. Clearly, menin appears to play a role in controlling cellular proliferation.

Menin also is involved in multiple cell signaling pathways. Menin interacts with the Smad family of proteins to inhibit the transforming growth factor-β (TGF-β) and bone morphogenetic protein-2 (BMP-2) signaling pathways [28–30]. Menin also may be involved in the Wnt signaling pathway through interactions with the transcription factor β-catenin. Interestingly, Wnt signaling stimulates pancreatic islet

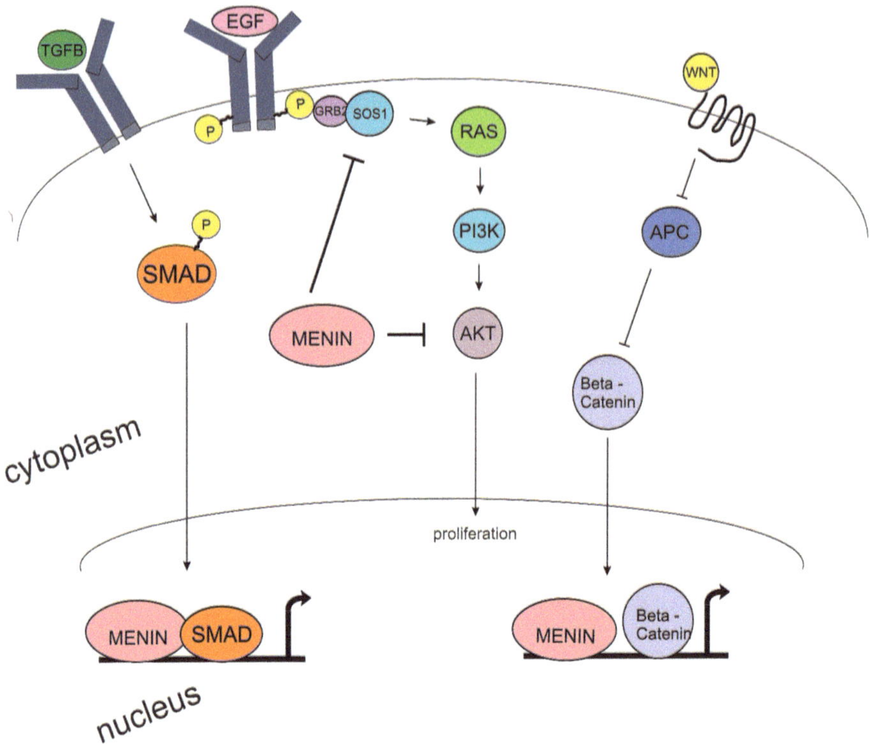

Fig. 2.1 Menin regulates multiple signaling pathways in the cell

β-cell proliferation. Over-expression of menin decreases nuclear β-catenin in part by directly binding and excluding it from the nucleus [31]. In contrast to that, menin also appears to be needed to interact with β-catenin for Wnt signaling in rodent islet tumor cells [32]. Although certainly interesting given the role of Wnt signaling in β-cell proliferation, the exact role of menin in the Wnt signaling pathway still remains to be elucidated.

In addition to roles in proliferation, genomic stability, and cell cycle regulation, menin also plays a role in epigenetic regulation of gene expression through histone methylation and acetylation. Menin is part of the mixed lineage leukemia (MLL) histone methyltransferase complex. Menin binds to MLL and mediates the H3K4 methyltransferase activity promoting histone H3 lysine 4 trimethylation which is linked to transcriptional activation [33–35]. As part of the MLL complex, menin is involved in the regulation of the homeobox genes and increasing expression of cyclin-dependent kinase inhibitors, p27 (*CDKN1B*) and p18 (*CDKN2C*) [33, 36–38]. In addition, menin may mediate the repression of genes targeted by JunD through recruitment of the histone deacetylase (HDAC) complex to suppress transcriptional activity [39, 40]. Finally, menin has been shown to interact with suppressor of variegation 3-9 homolog family protein (SUV39H1) to mediate H3K4 methylation and silence transcriptional activity of target genes [41].

Menin has been shown to be involved in neuroendocrine cell development and function. Menin regulates proliferation in normal pancreatic islet cells [33, 42, 43]. *Men1*−/− mice are embryonic lethal [44]. *Men1*+/− mice develop pancreatic islet cell hyperplasia and multiple endocrine tumors with a prolonged latency [45]. Conditional *Men1* gene knockout in pancreatic β-cells results in the development of insulinomas with full penetrance, and none of the tumors become poorly differentiated [46, 47]. These data suggest that *Men1* mutations are drivers for PNET formation; however, additional mutations are needed to convert PNETs into high-grade tumors. Recently, menin ablation in mouse pancreatic islet cells was shown to enhance Hedgehog signaling, a pro-proliferative and oncogenic pathway [48]. These studies demonstrate that menin directly interacts with protein arginine methyltransferase 5 (PRMT5), a negative regulator of gene transcription. Menin recruits PRMT5 to the promoter of the *Gas1* gene, a crucial factor for binding of Sonic Hedgehog (Shh) ligand to its receptor. This binding increases the repressive histone 4 arginine dimethylation (H4R3m2s) mark at the *Gas1* promoter thereby suppressing expression of *Gas1* [48]. Menin mutant mice have reduced binding to PRMT5 and therefore fail to provide the repressive H4R3m2s mark at *Gas1* promoter, resulting in elevated gene expression and increased Hedgehog signaling. In mice, pharmacological inhibition of Hedgehog signaling reduces proliferation of insulinoma cells [48]. This novel finding suggests that menin-PRMT5 interaction epigenetically suppresses Hedgehog signaling, making this pathway a potential target for treatment of *MEN1* mutated tumors.

2.7 von Hippel–Lindau Disease

von Hippel–Lindau disease (vHL) is an autosomal dominant hereditary cancer syndrome with an incidence in the United States of 1 in 32,000 and penetrance over 90 % by age 65 [49]. vHL is caused by germline mutations in the *VHL* gene and associate with several benign and malignant tumor types including hemangioblastomas of the central nervous system (brain, spinal cord, and retina), renal cysts and clear cell renal cell carcinoma (RCC), endolymphatic sac tumors, epididymal cystadenomas, pheochromocytomas (PCC), and pancreatic cysts and PNETs. PNETs occur in 9–17 % of patients with vHL [50–52]. vHL-associated PNETs display differential expression of genes related to angiogenesis and hypoxia-inducible factor signaling compared to sporadic PNETs [53]. Meta-analysis of 1,442 patients with vHL found that of 420 patients who were assessed for pancreatic lesions, 60 % had pancreatic masses, 47 % of which were simple cysts [51]. PNETs were found in 15 % of patients and only 2 % of those were malignant and so vHL-associated PNETs are associated with very different prognosis (improved) than sporadic PNETs [51]. vHL-associated PNETs are nonfunctional. Notably, patients with vHL often have multiple pancreatic cysts and masses. In patients with vHL, surgical removal of PNETs is recommended for pancreatic lesions over 3 cm, as this size cutoff is associated with more aggressive disease. Further indicators of malignant potential are quickly growing tumors and those associated with inherited mutations in the third exon of *VHL* [50].

2.8 *VHL* Gene and Mutations

The *VHL* gene is located on chromosome 3p25-26 and contains three exons which span 639 bp and encodes for two VHL proteins, one full-length 213 amino acids, and a smaller protein that lacks the first 53 amino acids. *VHL* is a tumor suppressor gene and most vHL-associated tumors show LOH of the wild-type allele as the second hit. Over 1,000 mutations in the *VHL* gene have been reported to date, which range across the gene and include missense, nonsense, and insertion/deletion mutations [54]. Genotype-phenotype correlations with *VHL* mutations have been well documented. Patients with type 1 vHL disease have a lower risk of developing PCC and a higher risk of RCC and other manifestations of vHL; they tend to have truncating mutations or exonic deletions. Patients with type 2 vHL disease tend to have missense mutations in the *VHL* gene, which are associated with much greater penetrance of PCC [55, 56]. Type 2 disease is further stratified into type 2A, which has a lower risk of clear cell RCC; type 2b, which is associated with a high risk of all manifestations of vHL; and type 2C, which is associated only with PCC. PNETs are associated with mutations throughout the *VHL* gene, but the development of metastatic disease appears to be higher in association with mutations in exon 3 [50].

In contrast to *MEN1*, somatic *VHL* point mutations in sporadic PNETs are rarely observed [20, 57]. Rather, up to 25 % of sporadic PNETs have been shown to have inactivation of *VHL* through promoter hypermethylation or gene deletion [57]. The presence of *VHL* methylation or deletions in sporadic PNETs has been suggested to be associated with worsened outcome [57].

2.9 VHL Protein

The VHL protein forms a complex with elongin B, elongin C, RBx 1 and Cul2 which has ubiquitin ligase E3 activity [58]. The major function of the VHL protein is to regulate the hypoxia-inducible transcription factors (HIF1α and HIF2α). Under normoxic conditions, VHL binds to the hydroxyproline residue on the HIFs targeting them for ubiquitination and proteosomal degradation [59]. Under hypoxic conditions, or if there is a mutation in *VHL*, this interaction cannot take place, resulting in the loss of ubiquitination of HIFα and thus allowing it to complex with a ubiquitous nuclear transporter HIF1β, also known as ARNT [58, 60]. In hypoxia situations, there is massive upregulation of over 100 genes now known to be induced because of activation by the transcription factors HIF1α and HIF2α [61, 62]. The activation of these target pathways serves to enhance tumorigenesis and includes genes involved in angiogenesis, glucose metabolism, cell survival, and cell migration/invasion properties [61, 62]. Although the consensus binding site for these transcription factors is the same, the factors themselves have overlapping, but not identical sets of target genes.

The VHL protein also has HIF-independent functions relevant to tumor development. VHL appears to be required for extracellular matrix assembly including binding to fibronectin and hydroxyl collagen IV-α2 [63, 64] and regulating some integrin functions for cellular adhesions [65]. In addition, VHL has been shown to directly bind p53, and the phosphorylation of VHL by checkpoint kinase 2 (Chk2) promotes transactivation of p53, resulting in apoptosis [66, 67]. VHL also promotes the inhibitory phosphorylation of NF-κB agonist CARD9, which leads to a decrease in NF-κB activity [68].

2.10 Neurofibromatosis Type 1

Neurofibromatosis type 1 (NF1), also called von Recklinghausen's disease, is an autosomal dominant disorder caused by inactivating mutations in the tumor suppressor gene, *NF1*. NF1 occurs in 1 in 3,000 individuals worldwide. The diagnosis is made based on clinical criteria. Patients must have at least two of the following features: six or more café-au-lait macules (at least 0.5 cm in prepubertal patients and 1.5 cm in postpubertal patients), two or more cutaneous neurofibromas or a single plexiform neurofibroma, inguinal or axillary freckling, two or more Lisch nodules (benign iris hamartomas), optic nerve glioma, dysplasia of the long bones, and a first-degree relative with NF1 [69]. Several cancers have been associated with NF1 at a higher frequency than the general population, including malignant peripheral nerve sheath tumors, gastrointestinal stromal tumors, chronic myeloid leukemia, and PNETs [70–72].

Numerous case reports of PNETs associated with NF1 are found in the literature; up to 10 % of NF1 patients are described as having PNETs. The most frequent NF1-associated PNET is the somatostatinoma. NF1-associated somatostatinomas more often are found in the duodenum rather than the pancreas [73]. Up to 48 % of duodenal somatostatinomas have been reported to be associated with NF1 [71, 73]. In one of the largest case series including 26 NF1 patients with somatostatinomas, the patients were more often female than male and ranged in age from 21 to 70 years old [74]. Interestingly, NF1-associated somatostatinomas infrequently present with symptoms of somatostatin syndrome because the tumors are less likely to hypersecrete hormones compared to sporadic duodenal somatostatinomas or pancreatic somatostatinomas [73]. Instead, these tumors tend to present with obstructive symptoms such as jaundice, weight loss, and abdominal pain. In other aspects, NF1-associated duodenal tumors are similar to sporadic tumors with both types having frequent psammoma bodies on pathologic examination and less frequent metastases compared to pancreatic somatostatinomas [73].

2.11 *NF1* Gene and Protein

The *NF1* gene is large, spanning 360 kb and over 60 exons located on chromosome 17q11.2. There are no hot spots for mutations and no genotype/phenotype correlations. No specific mutations are associated with PNET development. Up to 50 % of NF1 patients arise from a de novo mutation, and interestingly, there is variable penetrance and expressivity of the disease even in patients with the same mutation [70]. The protein neurofibromin is composed of 2,818 amino acids, and the most well-characterized function of this large protein is as a GTPase which inactivates Ras to inhibit the MAPK signaling pathway. When *NF1* is mutated, there is constitutive activation of Ras and hence the downstream MAPK, PI3K, and mTOR pathways, leading to uncontrolled cellular growth and differentiation [75–77]. *NF1* has been found to be mutated in a multiplicity of tumor types, ranging from glioblastoma multiforme to melanoma, lung, ovarian, and bladder cancers among others based on data from the Cancer Genome Atlas.

2.12 Tuberous Sclerosis Complex

Tuberous Sclerosis Complex (TSC) is another autosomal dominant disease with prevalence of 1 in 6–10 thousand individuals [78]. The clinical manifestations include abnormalities of the brain (cortical tubers, subependymal nodules, seizure disorders, developmental delay), skin (facial angiofibromas, ungual and periungual fibromas, hypomelanotic macules), kidney (renal angiomyolipomas, cysts), lungs (lymphangiomyomatosis), and eyes (hamartomas) [78]. Two-thirds of patients have no family history of TSC and are thought to be due to de novo mutations, particularly in *TSC2*. Eighty to 85 % of patients meeting clinical criteria for TSC are found to have mutations in one of two genes, *TSC1* and *TSC2* [79, 80]. No other genes are thought to be associated with TSC; rather it is thought that the mutations may not be detectable in some cases due to issues such as somatic mosaicism or being outside the region interrogated by clinical testing (e.g., promoter region). *TSC1* is located on chromosome 9q34 and spans 55 kb of DNA encoding 23 exons. *TSC2* is located on chromosome 16p13 and spans 40 kb encoding 41 exons. The gene products are hamartin and tuberin, respectively, which share no homology. These two proteins dimerize to control cellular proliferation through the PI3 kinase/mTOR pathway [81]. Truncating mutations span both genes without particular hot spots, although mutations in *TSC2* are more common in both familial and sporadic cases [82]. Missense mutations in *TSC2* tend to cluster in the GTPase-activating protein-binding domain and are rare in *TSC1*. Large genomic deletions also are more frequent in *TSC2* than in *TSC1* [83]. PNETs in TSC are extremely rare with only a handful of cases reported in the literature with most having mutations in *TSC2* when tested [84]. The tumors tend to be well differentiated and can be secretory.

2.13 Somatic Genetic Mutations in PNETs

Candidate gene approaches to identify somatic mutations in PNETs have been performed in small studies with variable results. Activating mutations in exon 3 of *β-catenin* were described in 37 % of gastrointestinal NETs [85] but not in PNETs [86].

Table 2.2 Common somatic mutations in PNETs

Gene	Loci	Protein	Function
MEN1	11q13.1	Menin	Regulates cellular proliferation
			Role in genomic stability
			Role in epigenetic regulation
DAXX	6q21.3	Death-domain-associated protein	Histone H3.3 chaperone
ATRX	Xq21.1	Alpha thalassemia/mental retardation syndrome X-linked protein	Member of the SWI-SNF family of chromatin remodeling proteins
PTEN	10q23.3	Phosphatidylinositol-3,4,5-trisphosphate 3-phosphatase	Phosphatase which preferentially dephosphorylates phosphoinositide substrates
			Key modulator of the AKT-mTOR signaling pathway
TSC2	16p13.3	Tuberin	Dimerizes with hamartin to control cellular proliferation through the PI3K/mTOR pathway

PTEN, *KRAS*, *TP53*, and *CDKN2A* are rarely mutated in PNETs [87–92]. One small study suggested that loss of PTEN expression by immunohistochemistry correlated with advanced tumor stage [93]. Another small study showed that although no point mutations were found in *CDKN2A*, the gene was homozygously deleted in 42 % and methylated in 58 % of gastrinomas and nonfunctioning PNETs [94]. Several small studies found no mutations in *RET*, *BRAF*, and *SMAD3* [95–98]. One small study did find *DPC4*/*SMAD4* mutations in a high percentage of sporadic PNETs [99], but this was not confirmed in subsequent larger studies [89, 100].

Massively parallel sequencing studies on PNETs have confirmed some of the previously known somatically mutated genes in PNETs and also have identified novel genes involved in tumorigenesis (Table 2.2). Whole-exome sequencing (WES) of ten advanced PNETs identified 157 somatic mutations in 149 genes with an average mutation rate of 16 mutations per tumor [19]. This low number of somatic mutations reflects the often indolent nature of PNETs compared to other more aggressive carcinomas which often have a median of 44 non-silent somatic mutations per tumor [101]. The most frequently mutated genes in the discovery PNET set were selected to be sequenced in a validation set of 58 additional PNETs. In total, this study confirmed the most commonly somatically mutated gene in well-differentiated PNETs is *MEN1* (in 44 % of cases) [19]. Fifteen percent of PNETs had a mutation in one of the PI3K/mTOR signaling pathway genes including *TSC2* (in 8.8 % of cases) and *PTEN* (in 7.3 % of cases) as well as one tumor with a *PIK3CA* activating mutation. The fact that a significant percentage of PNETs have mutations in genes regulating the mTOR pathway is consistent with the observation that patients with PNETs respond to the mTOR inhibitor everolimus with improved progression-free survival [102]. Perhaps identifying patients with a somatic mutation in the mTOR pathway before treatment could serve as a biomarker to predict response to directed therapy with everolimus in the future.

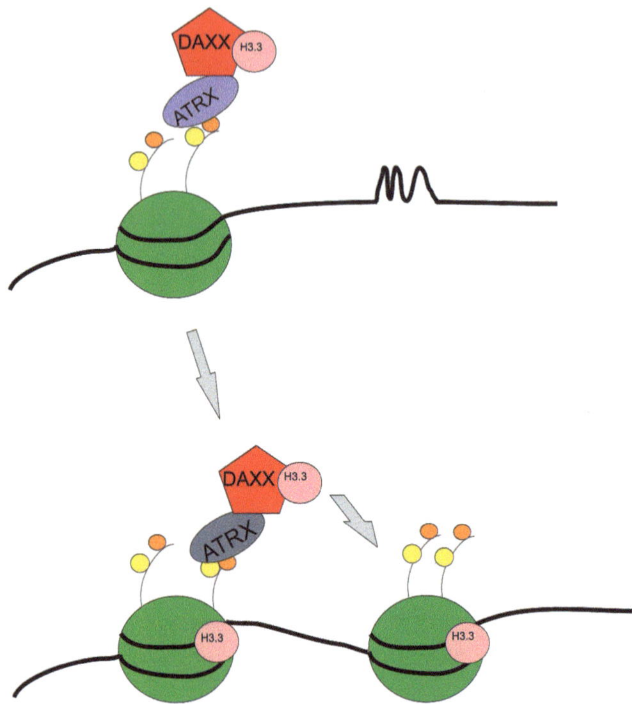

Fig. 2.2 Recruitment of ATRX/DAXX complex to heterochromatin with G4 DNA structures. The ATRX ADD domain binds with a histone H3 trimethylated Lys 9 and unmodified Lys 4. The ATRX binding partner DAXX recruits histone variant H3.3 and the complex deposits H3.3 into the nucleosome to maintain the DNA in the B form (*orange circle*, histone H3 K9me3; *yellow circle*, histone H3 K4me0)

WES also identified that the second most commonly identified somatic mutations are in the *DAXX/ATRX* complex (in 43 % of cases) which was not previously known to play a role in the biology of PNETs [19]. *DAXX* and *ATRX* are both part of the chromatin remodeling complex (Fig. 2.2). Mutations in either *DAXX* (death-domain-associated protein, in 25 % of cases) or *ATRX* (alpha thalassemia/mental retardation syndrome X-linked in 18 % of cases) were mutually exclusive with each other but sometimes demonstrate overlap with mutations in *MEN1* (in 23.5 % of cases) [19]. Interestingly, *DAXX/ATRX* mutations were associated with a statistically significant increase in overall survival, which improved further if there was an additional *MEN1* mutation [19]. These data should be interpreted with caution given the small numbers of tumors with *MEN1* and *DAXX/ATRX* mutations in the study. Nevertheless, these data are consistent with a study examining protein expression in well-differentiated PNETs versus poorly differentiated neuroendocrine carcinomas. In this study, DAXX and ATRX expression by immunohistochemistry (IHC) are mutually exclusively lost in 45 % of well-differentiated PNETs, similar to the mutation rate and pattern seen by WES, whereas p53 and Rb showed normal expression [103].

Conversely, p53 and Rb protein expression by IHC was altered in poorly differentiated neuroendocrine carcinomas compared with well-differentiated PNETs, whereas expression of ATRX and DAXX was the same in both tumor sets [103]. However, recently a larger study of 149 PNETs had contrasting results with the absence of DAXX/ATRX staining by IHC associated with chromosomal instability and decreased relapse-free survival in patients with PNETs [104]. Given the differing results, additional studies need to be performed to understand the true association of *DAXX/ATRX* mutations with prognosis in PNETs. Nonetheless, mutations in this complex appear to play a significant role in PNET tumorigenesis, although the mechanism is still being elucidated.

The *ATRX* gene is located on the X chromosome at Xq21.1, has 36 exons, and encodes a 2,492 amino acid protein. Germline *ATRX* mutations lead to ATRX syndrome in which patients develop a neurodevelopmental condition with various degrees of gonadal dysgenesis and alpha thalassemia [105]. Similar to other X-linked disorders, female patients with germline *ATRX* mutations are generally unaffected or only mildly affected as they exhibit skewed X chromosomal inactivation patterns; hence the syndrome is predominantly seen in males [106]. ATRX is a large nuclear protein with a C-terminal ATPase/DNA helicase domain making it part of the SWI-SNF family of chromatin remodeling proteins. The N-terminal domain has a DNA-binding domain which recognizes the methylation status of lysine residues on histone 3 which typically denotes inactive heterochromatin, including telomeric and pericentric regions. ATRX has also been associated with G-quadruplex formations of DNA which prevent DNA and RNA polymerases from functioning [107]. ATRX is thought to play a role in resolving G-quadruplex DNA formations, thereby promoting gene expression. ATRX depletion leads to loss of structural integrity at telomeres which have high concentration of G-quadruplex formation, while treatment with G-quadruplex-stabilizing agents in ATRX-depleted cells causes DNA damage at telomeres, such as chromosomal end-to-end fusions and telomere deletions [108]. ATRX-deficient mice have defective chromosomal cohesion during mitosis, increased sensitivity to agents that induce replicative stress, and increased p53-mediated apoptosis in response to DNA damage [108]. These studies suggest ATRX serves to help maintain genomic integrity.

Interestingly, the germline mutations associated with ATRX syndrome differ from the somatic mutations found in PNET tumors. Fifty percent of germline mutations are in exons 8–10 in the DNA-binding domain and about 30 % are in exons 17–31 in the helicase domains [109]. Furthermore, the inherited ATRX mutations tend to be hypomorphic missense mutations rather than protein-truncating mutations which lead to loss of protein through nonsense-mediated decay as seen with the somatic mutations. This finding is not surprising since ATRX appears to be essential for life as mice deficient in ATRX are embryonic lethal [110].

DAXX is located on chromosome 6q21.3, has eight exons, and encodes a 688 amino acid protein. DAXX also is a nuclear protein and functions as a histone H3.3 chaperone. The ATRX-DAXX complex assembles H3.3 into nucleosomes and, therefore, is implicated in chromatin stabilization [111–113]. ATRX recruits DAXX to bring H3.3 to telomeres and pericentric heterochromatin [113]. It is hypothesized that disruption of this function leads to tumorigenesis by disrupting regulation of telomeres as protein loss of DAXX or ATRX is correlated with alternative lengthening of telomeres (ALT), a telomerase-independent mechanism of telomere lengthening [114]. Alternative lengthening of telomeres through DNA recombination has been shown in 61 % of PNETs in one study and 19 of those 25 tumors had mutations in either *ATRX* or *DAXX* [114]. Alternative lengthening of telomeres was seen in all *DAXX/ATRX* mutated tumors in the whole-exome sequencing study of non-MEN1-associated PNETs [19]. In MEN1-associated PNETs, only a small subset had *DAXX/ATRX* mutations, but all of the mutation-positive tumors had the ALT phenotype [115]. Interestingly, in a study of multiple cancer types including PNETs, all tumors which had *ATRX* mutations were ALT positive by a telomere FISH assay [116]. *ATRX* mutations are not restricted to neuroendocrine tumors but are found in other tumor types as well including gliomas. The ATRX/DAXX complex appears to be critical for genomic integrity, and disruption of this process appears to lead to tumorigenesis. Nevertheless, the precise mechanism of ATRX/DAXX dysfunction in pancreatic neuroendocrine tumorigenesis is still being elucidated.

2.14 Expression Profiling

Several studies have examined expression profiling in PNETs and have highlighted specific altered cellular pathways in subsets of tumors. Comparing nonfunctioning well-differentiated PNETs to pancreatic islet cell samples, very few differentially expressed genes were identified [117]. However, when examining differences in the expression profiles of metastatic and non-metastatic PNETs, there was increased expression of genes involved in growth regulation, cholesterol homeostasis, osmotic regulation, and hypoxia-inducible factors and under-expression of genes involved in the cell cycle and DNA damage response in the metastatic subset [118]. Another study of PNETs with and without metastases showed that metastatic tumors had higher expression in genes involved in angiogenesis, signal transduction through tyrosine kinases, and calcium-dependent cell signaling [119]. Malignant tumors also showed activation of insulin-like growth factor-signaling cascade [118, 119]. Interestingly, another study comparing nonfunctioning PNETs (primary tumors and associated metastases) to islet cell preparations found that similar expression patterns between primary tumors and associated metastatic tumor, suggesting malignant potential, may be acquired at an early stage [120]. *ANG2* (*angiopoietin-2*) has been suggested as a potential molecular marker for malignancy as it was over-expressed in a microarray study in 89 % of nonfunctional PNETs compared with 22 % of normal pancreas samples [121]. Another potential marker for worsened disease-free and overall survival is co-downregulation of *PTEN* and *TSC2* [122]. *RUNX1T1* is under-expressed in well-differentiated metastatic primary PNETs relative to non-metastatic primaries and, therefore, could represent a possible biomarker for prediction of metastases [123]. Most of these studies have been done in small sample sets, and further validation is needed to confirm these genes as possible biomarkers for metastases and survival.

2.15 Copy Number Aberrations

Array-based comparative genomic hybridization (aCGH) studies have shown that PNETs have multiple chromosomal alterations. Not surprisingly, genetic alterations accumulate during tumor progression and increase in concert with tumor volume and stage [124]. In addition, more copy number gains and losses are found in metastatic disease compared to benign tumors [124, 125]. Loss of chromosome 1 and 11q and gains of 9q appear to be early events because these alterations are seen in many small tumors under 2 cm [124]. The *MEN1* gene is located on chromosome 11q, so loss of this region early in tumorigenesis is not surprising. Potential genes of interest in the other commonly disrupted chromosomal regions included tumor suppressor genes on chromosome 1 including *TP73* and *RIZ* and oncogenes on chromosome 9q included *ABL* and *VAV2*. In one study of 25 PNETs, 68 % of tumors had gain on chromosome 7 with the minimal overlapping region at 7q11.2 which contains potential genes of interest including *MET* and *EGFR* [126]. Loss of chromosome 3pq and 6pq and gains of 14q, 17pq and 20q are associated with advanced stage and malignant behavior [124, 127]. In metastases, gains of chromosome 4pq, 5q, 7pq, and 17q and losses of 11pq, 10p, 3p, and 6q are seen often [125]. Insulinomas have fewer alterations than other PNETs and often have gains of chromosome 9q32 [124–127].

2.16 Epigenetics

Gene-specific analysis has identified some genes commonly epigenetically silenced in PNETs. *RASSF1A* is a tumor suppressor gene located on chromosome 3q21 and frequently methylated in several cancer types. In PNETs, *RASSF1A* promoter methylation has been reported in as high as 75–83 % of tumors and correlates with larger tumors and the presence of metastatic disease; however, methylation of *RASSF1A* also has been found in adjacent normal tissue making the role for silencing this gene uncertain [128–131]. *CDKN2A* is a tumor suppressor gene located on chromosome 9p21 and encodes the p16 protein which regulates the cell cycle. *CDKN2A* is commonly silenced by promoter methylation in cancers including 10–58 % of PNETs and correlated with the presence of metastatic disease [91, 94, 129, 132, 133]. Methylation status of other genes has conflicting reports in various studies. The *MGMT* promoter was methylated in 40 % of 48 PNETs in one study [129] but in none of 11 PNETs in another study [133]. Similarly, *TIMP3* encoding an extracellular protease inhibitor, known to play a role in metastatic potential in cancers, was methylated in 44 % of functional PNETs [134] but not in insulinomas or nonfunctional PNETs [129, 134].

CpG island methylator phenotype (CIMP) is known to be associated with colorectal adenocarcinomas. In a series of neuroendocrine tumors, CIMP phenotype was found in 50 % of gastrinomas and up to 100 % of VIPomas and glucagonomas, all associated with high Ki67 proliferative index [135]. High promoter methylation in PNETs has been associated with higher-grade tumors, early recurrence, and worse prognosis with decreased survival [129, 135]. Future studies using massively parallel sequencing of the methylome may help to further elucidate the role of epigenetic methylation in PNET tumorigenesis.

2.17 Small Intestinal NETS

Massively parallel sequencing of small intestinal NETs (SINETs) identified a low number of somatic alterations similar to PNETs [136]. Banck et al. examined 48 ileal and small bowel carcinoid tumors grades 1 and 2 through whole-exome sequencing and found a total of 197 non-synonymous mutations and 14 splice-site mutations. No recurrent mutations were identified. In fact, only one gene was mutated in more than one tumor (*ABCC12* mutations in two of 48 tumors). Several known cancer-promoting genes were mutated in single cases including *BRAF*, *FANCD2*, *FGFR2*, *MEN1*, and *VHL* [136].

Somatic copy number analysis in the SINETs showed a low rate of copy number changes per tumor (average 21) suggesting relative genomic stability [136]. The pattern of gains and losses was consistent with previous studies using aCGH and SNP arrays [137, 138]. Copy number gains were found in *MTOR* (6 % of cases) and *SRC* (23 % of cases), whereas copy number loss was common in *SMAD4* tumor suppressor gene in 46 % of cases [136]. Interestingly, *SMAD4* is frequently mutated in pancreatic adenocarcinomas although not seen in PNETs [89, 100].

2.18 Summary and Future Directions

Given the poor prognosis associated with metastatic PNETs, it is essential to identify biomarkers for prediction of malignant potential and to identify novel targets for therapeutics to treat metastatic disease. Recently, our understanding of tumorigenesis in PNETs has expanded from studies focusing solely on the role of menin as a tumor suppressor to massively parallel sequencing studies identifying potential new drivers of tumorigenesis in PNETs. However, further work needs to be done to fully understand the mechanism of tumorigenesis behind the newly discovered somatically mutated genes to enable the development of therapeutics.

References

1. Lawrence B, Gustafsson BI, Chan A, Svejda B, Kidd M, Modlin IM. The epidemiology of gastroenteropancreatic neuroendocrine tumors. Endocrinol Metab Clin North Am. 2011;40(1):1–18, vii. Epub 2011/02/26.
2. Kimura W, Kuroda A, Morioka Y. Clinical pathology of endocrine tumors of the pancreas. Analysis of autopsy cases. Dig Dis Sci. 1991;36(7):933–42. Epub 1991/07/01.

3. Franko J, Feng W, Yip L, Genovese E, Moser AJ. Non-functional neuroendocrine carcinoma of the pancreas: incidence, tumor biology, and outcomes in 2,158 patients. J Gastrointest Surg. 2010;14(3):541–8. Epub 2009/12/10.
4. Bilimoria KY, Tomlinson JS, Merkow RP, Stewart AK, Ko CY, Talamonti MS, et al. Clinicopathologic features and treatment trends of pancreatic neuroendocrine tumors: analysis of 9,821 patients. J Gastrointest Surg. 2007;11(11):1460–7. discussion 7–9. Epub 2007/09/12.
5. Frilling A, Sotiropoulos GC, Li J, Kornasiewicz O, Plockinger U. Multimodal management of neuroendocrine liver metastases. HPB (Oxford). 2010;12(6):361–79. Epub 2010/07/29.
6. Khasraw M, Gill A, Harrington T, Pavlakis N, Modlin I. Management of advanced neuroendocrine tumors with hepatic metastasis. J Clin Gastroenterol. 2009;43(9):838–47. Epub 2009/08/06.
7. Meeker A, Heaphy C. Gastroenteropancreatic endocrine tumors. Mol Cell Endocrinol. 2014;386(1–2):101–20. Epub 2013/08/03.
8. Oberg K, Knigge U, Kwekkeboom D, Perren A. Neuroendocrine gastro-entero-pancreatic tumors: ESMO Clinical Practice Guidelines for diagnosis, treatment and follow-up. Ann Oncol. 2012;23 Suppl 7:vii124–30. Epub 2012/11/20.
9. Kunz PL, Reidy-Lagunes D, Anthony LB, Bertino EM, Brendtro K, Chan JA, et al. Consensus guidelines for the management and treatment of neuroendocrine tumors. Pancreas. 2013;42(4):557–77. Epub 2013/04/18.
10. Thakker RV, Newey PJ, Walls GV, Bilezikian J, Dralle H, Ebeling PR, et al. Clinical practice guidelines for multiple endocrine neoplasia type 1 (MEN1). J Clin Endocrinol Metab. 2012;97(9):2990–3011. Epub 2012/06/23.
11. Brandi ML, Gagel RF, Angeli A, Bilezikian JP, Beck-Peccoz P, Bordi C, et al. Guidelines for diagnosis and therapy of MEN type 1 and type 2. J Clin Endocrinol Metab. 2001;86(12):5658–71. Epub 2001/12/12.
12. Scheithauer BW, Laws Jr ER, Kovacs K, Horvath E, Randall RV, Carney JA. Pituitary adenomas of the multiple endocrine neoplasia type I syndrome. Semin Diagn Pathol. 1987;4(3):205–11. Epub 1987/08/01.
13. Metz DC, Jensen RT. Gastrointestinal neuroendocrine tumors: pancreatic endocrine tumors. Gastroenterology. 2008;135(5):1469–92. Epub 2008/08/16.
14. Marx S, Spiegel AM, Skarulis MC, Doppman JL, Collins FS, Liotta LA. Multiple endocrine neoplasia type 1: clinical and genetic topics. Ann Intern Med. 1998;129(6):484–94. Epub 1998/09/12.
15. Chandrasekharappa SC, Guru SC, Manickam P, Olufemi SE, Collins FS, Emmert-Buck MR, et al. Positional cloning of the gene for multiple endocrine neoplasia-type 1. Science. 1997;276(5311):404–7. Epub 1997/04/18.
16. Agarwal SK, Kester MB, Debelenko LV, Heppner C, Emmert-Buck MR, Skarulis MC, et al. Germline mutations of the MEN1 gene in familial multiple endocrine neoplasia type 1 and related states. Hum Mol Genet. 1997;6(7):1169–75. Epub 1997/07/01.
17. Lemos MC, Thakker RV. Multiple endocrine neoplasia type 1 (MEN1): analysis of 1336 mutations reported in the first decade following identification of the gene. Hum Mutat. 2008;29(1):22–32. Epub 2007/09/20.
18. Bassett JH, Forbes SA, Pannett AA, Lloyd SE, Christie PT, Wooding C, et al. Characterization of mutations in patients with multiple endocrine neoplasia type 1. Am J Hum Genet. 1998;62(2):232–44. Epub 1998/04/16.
19. Jiao Y, Shi C, Edil BH, de Wilde RF, Klimstra DS, Maitra A, et al. DAXX/ATRX, MEN1, and mTOR pathway genes are frequently altered in pancreatic neuroendocrine tumors. Science. 2011;331(6021):1199–203. Epub 2011/01/22.
20. Moore PS, Missiaglia E, Antonello D, Zamo A, Zamboni G, Corleto V, et al. Role of disease-causing genes in sporadic pancreatic endocrine tumors: MEN1 and VHL. Genes Chromosomes Cancer. 2001;32(2):177–81. Epub 2001/09/11.
21. Corbo V, Dalai I, Scardoni M, Barbi S, Beghelli S, Bersani S, et al. MEN1 in pancreatic endocrine tumors: analysis of gene and protein status in 169 sporadic neoplasms reveals

alterations in the vast majority of cases. Endocr Relat Cancer. 2010;17(3):771–83. Epub 2010/06/23.

22. Goebel SU, Heppner C, Burns AL, Marx SJ, Spiegel AM, Zhuang Z, et al. Genotype/phenotype correlation of multiple endocrine neoplasia type 1 gene mutations in sporadic gastrinomas. J Clin Endocrinol Metab. 2000;85(1):116–23. Epub 2000/01/14.
23. Gortz B, Roth J, Krahenmann A, de Krijger RR, Muletta-Feurer S, Rutimann K, et al. Mutations and allelic deletions of the MEN1 gene are associated with a subset of sporadic endocrine pancreatic and neuroendocrine tumors and not restricted to foregut neoplasms. Am J Pathol. 1999;154(2):429–36. Epub 1999/02/23.
24. Guru SC, Goldsmith PK, Burns AL, Marx SJ, Spiegel AM, Collins FS, et al. Menin, the product of the MEN1 gene, is a nuclear protein. Proc Natl Acad Sci U S A. 1998;95(4):1630–4. Epub 1998/03/21.
25. Lin SY, Elledge SJ. Multiple tumor suppressor pathways negatively regulate telomerase. Cell. 2003;113(7):881–9. Epub 2003/07/03.
26. Wang Y, Ozawa A, Zaman S, Prasad NB, Chandrasekharappa SC, Agarwal SK, et al. The tumor suppressor protein menin inhibits AKT activation by regulating its cellular localization. Cancer Res. 2011;71(2):371–82. Epub 2010/12/04.
27. Heppner C, Bilimoria KY, Agarwal SK, Kester M, Whitty LJ, Guru SC, et al. The tumor suppressor protein menin interacts with NF-kappaB proteins and inhibits NF-kappaB-mediated transactivation. Oncogene. 2001;20(36):4917–25. Epub 2001/08/30.
28. Sowa H, Kaji H, Hendy GN, Canaff L, Komori T, Sugimoto T, et al. Menin is required for bone morphogenetic protein 2- and transforming growth factor beta-regulated osteoblastic differentiation through interaction with Smads and Runx2. J Biol Chem. 2004;279(39):40267–75. Epub 2004/05/20.
29. Sowa H, Kaji H, Canaff L, Hendy GN, Tsukamoto T, Yamaguchi T, et al. Inactivation of menin, the product of the multiple endocrine neoplasia type 1 gene, inhibits the commitment of multipotential mesenchymal stem cells into the osteoblast lineage. J Biol Chem. 2003;278(23):21058–69. Epub 2003/03/22.
30. Kaji H, Canaff L, Lebrun JJ, Goltzman D, Hendy GN. Inactivation of menin, a Smad3-interacting protein, blocks transforming growth factor type beta signaling. Proc Natl Acad Sci U S A. 2001;98(7):3837–42. Epub 2001/03/29.
31. Cao Y, Liu R, Jiang X, Lu J, Jiang J, Zhang C, et al. Nuclear-cytoplasmic shuttling of menin regulates nuclear translocation of {beta}-catenin. Mol Cell Biol. 2009;29(20):5477–87. Epub 2009/08/05.
32. Chen G, A J, Wang M, Farley S, Lee LY, Lee LC, et al. Menin promotes the Wnt signaling pathway in pancreatic endocrine cells. Mol Cancer Res. 2008;6(12):1894–907. Epub 2008/12/17.
33. Karnik SK, Hughes CM, Gu X, Rozenblatt-Rosen O, McLean GW, Xiong Y, et al. Menin regulates pancreatic islet growth by promoting histone methylation and expression of genes encoding p27Kip1 and p18INK4c. Proc Natl Acad Sci U S A. 2005;102(41):14659–64. Epub 2005/10/01.
34. Murai MJ, Chruszcz M, Reddy G, Grembecka J, Cierpicki T. Crystal structure of menin reveals binding site for mixed lineage leukemia (MLL) protein. J Biol Chem. 2011;286(36):31742–8. Epub 2011/07/16.
35. Yokoyama A, Somervaille TC, Smith KS, Rozenblatt-Rosen O, Meyerson M, Cleary ML. The menin tumor suppressor protein is an essential oncogenic cofactor for MLL-associated leukemogenesis. Cell. 2005;123(2):207–18. Epub 2005/10/22.
36. Agarwal SK, Jothi R. Genome-wide characterization of menin-dependent H3K4me3 reveals a specific role for menin in the regulation of genes implicated in MEN1-like tumors. PLoS One. 2012;7(5):e37952. Epub 2012/06/06.
37. Yokoyama A, Wang Z, Wysocka J, Sanyal M, Aufiero DJ, Kitabayashi I, et al. Leukemia proto-oncoprotein MLL forms a SET1-like histone methyltransferase complex with menin to regulate Hox gene expression. Mol Cell Biol. 2004;24(13):5639–49. Epub 2004/06/17.
38. Wu T, Hua X. Menin represses tumorigenesis via repressing cell proliferation. Am J Cancer Res. 2011;1(6):726–39. Epub 2011/10/22.

39. Kim H, Lee JE, Cho EJ, Liu JO, Youn HD. Menin, a tumor suppressor, represses JunD-mediated transcriptional activity by association with an mSin3A-histone deacetylase complex. Cancer Res. 2003;63(19):6135–9. Epub 2003/10/16.
40. Kim H, Lee JE, Kim BY, Cho EJ, Kim ST, Youn HD. Menin represses JunD transcriptional activity in protein kinase C theta-mediated Nur77 expression. Exp Mol Med. 2005;37(5):466–75. Epub 2005/11/03.
41. Yang YJ, Song TY, Park J, Lee J, Lim J, Jang H, et al. Menin mediates epigenetic regulation via histone H3 lysine 9 methylation. Cell Death Dis. 2013;4:e583. Epub 2013/04/13.
42. Schnepp RW, Chen YX, Wang H, Cash T, Silva A, Diehl JA, et al. Mutation of tumor suppressor gene Men1 acutely enhances proliferation of pancreatic islet cells. Cancer Res. 2006;66(11):5707–15. Epub 2006/06/03.
43. Zhang H, Li W, Wang Q, Wang X, Li F, Zhang C, et al. Glucose-mediated repression of menin promotes pancreatic beta-cell proliferation. Endocrinology. 2012;153(2):602–11. Epub 2011/12/15.
44. Bertolino P, Radovanovic I, Casse H, Aguzzi A, Wang ZQ, Zhang CX. Genetic ablation of the tumor suppressor menin causes lethality at mid-gestation with defects in multiple organs. Mech Dev. 2003;120(5):549–60. Epub 2003/06/05.
45. Crabtree JS, Scacheri PC, Ward JM, Garrett-Beal L, Emmert-Buck MR, Edgemon KA, et al. A mouse model of multiple endocrine neoplasia, type 1, develops multiple endocrine tumors. Proc Natl Acad Sci U S A. 2001;98(3):1118–23. Epub 2001/02/07.
46. Crabtree JS, Scacheri PC, Ward JM, McNally SR, Swain GP, Montagna C, et al. Of mice and MEN1: Insulinomas in a conditional mouse knockout. Mol Cell Biol. 2003;23(17):6075–85. Epub 2003/08/15.
47. Bertolino P, Tong WM, Herrera PL, Casse H, Zhang CX, Wang ZQ. Pancreatic beta-cell-specific ablation of the multiple endocrine neoplasia type 1 (MEN1) gene causes full penetrance of insulinoma development in mice. Cancer Res. 2003;63(16):4836–41. Epub 2003/08/28.
48. Gurung B, Feng Z, Iwamoto DV, Thiel A, Jin G, Fan CM, et al. Menin epigenetically represses Hedgehog signaling in MEN1 tumor syndrome. Cancer Res. 2013;73(8):2650–8. Epub 2013/04/13.
49. Maher ER, Iselius L, Yates JR, Littler M, Benjamin C, Harris R, et al. Von Hippel-Lindau disease: a genetic study. J Med Genet. 1991;28(7):443–7. Epub 1991/07/01.
50. Blansfield JA, Choyke L, Morita SY, Choyke PL, Pingpank JF, Alexander HR, et al. Clinical, genetic and radiographic analysis of 108 patients with von Hippel-Lindau disease (VHL) manifested by pancreatic neuroendocrine neoplasms (PNETs). Surgery. 2007;142(6):814–8; discussion 8 e1–2. Epub 2007/12/08.
51. Charlesworth M, Verbeke CS, Falk GA, Walsh M, Smith AM, Morris-Stiff G. Pancreatic lesions in von Hippel-Lindau disease? A systematic review and meta-synthesis of the literature. J Gastrointest Surg. 2012;16(7):1422–8. Epub 2012/03/01.
52. Hammel PR, Vilgrain V, Terris B, Penfornis A, Sauvanet A, Correas JM, et al. Pancreatic involvement in von Hippel-Lindau disease. The Groupe Francophone d'Etude de la Maladie de von Hippel-Lindau. Gastroenterology. 2000;119(4):1087–95. Epub 2000/10/21.
53. Speisky D, Duces A, Bieche I, Rebours V, Hammel P, Sauvanet A, et al. Molecular profiling of pancreatic neuroendocrine tumors in sporadic and Von Hippel-Lindau patients. Clin Cancer Res. 2012;18(10):2838–49. Epub 2012/03/31.
54. Nordstrom-O'Brien M, van der Luijt RB, van Rooijen E, van den Ouweland AM, Majoor-Krakauer DF, Lolkema MP, et al. Genetic analysis of von Hippel-Lindau disease. Hum Mutat. 2010;31(5):521–37. Epub 2010/02/13.
55. Rechsteiner MP, von Teichman A, Nowicka A, Sulser T, Schraml P, Moch H. VHL gene mutations and their effects on hypoxia inducible factor HIFalpha: identification of potential driver and passenger mutations. Cancer Res. 2011;71(16):5500–11. Epub 2011/07/01.
56. Forman JR, Worth CL, Bickerton GR, Eisen TG, Blundell TL. Structural bioinformatics mutation analysis reveals genotype-phenotype correlations in von Hippel-Lindau disease and suggests molecular mechanisms of tumorigenesis. Proteins. 2009;77(1):84–96. Epub 2009/05/02.

57. Schmitt AM, Schmid S, Rudolph T, Anlauf M, Prinz C, Kloppel G, et al. VHL inactivation is an important pathway for the development of malignant sporadic pancreatic endocrine tumors. Endocr Relat Cancer. 2009;16(4):1219–27. Epub 2009/08/20.
58. Kaelin Jr WG. Molecular basis of the VHL hereditary cancer syndrome. Nat Rev Cancer. 2002;2(9):673–82. Epub 2002/09/05.
59. Min JH, Yang H, Ivan M, Gertler F, Kaelin Jr WG, Pavletich NP. Structure of an HIF-1alpha -pVHL complex: hydroxyproline recognition in signaling. Science. 2002;296(5574):1886–9. Epub 2002/05/11.
60. Wenger RH. Cellular adaptation to hypoxia: O2-sensing protein hydroxylases, hypoxia-inducible transcription factors, and O2-regulated gene expression. FASEB J. 2002; 16(10):1151–62. Epub 2002/08/03.
61. Hu CJ, Wang LY, Chodosh LA, Keith B, Simon MC. Differential roles of hypoxia-inducible factor 1alpha (HIF-1alpha) and HIF-2alpha in hypoxic gene regulation. Mol Cell Biol. 2003;23(24):9361–74. Epub 2003/12/04.
62. Hu CJ, Iyer S, Sataur A, Covello KL, Chodosh LA, Simon MC. Differential regulation of the transcriptional activities of hypoxia-inducible factor 1 alpha (HIF-1alpha) and HIF-2alpha in stem cells. Mol Cell Biol. 2006;26(9):3514–26. Epub 2006/04/14.
63. Ohh M, Yauch RL, Lonergan KM, Whaley JM, Stemmer-Rachamimov AO, Louis DN, et al. The von Hippel-Lindau tumor suppressor protein is required for proper assembly of an extracellular fibronectin matrix. Mol Cell. 1998;1(7):959–68. Epub 1998/07/04.
64. Kurban G, Duplan E, Ramlal N, Hudon V, Sado Y, Ninomiya Y, et al. Collagen matrix assembly is driven by the interaction of von Hippel-Lindau tumor suppressor protein with hydroxylated collagen IV alpha 2. Oncogene. 2008;27(7):1004–12. Epub 2007/08/19.
65. Esteban-Barragan MA, Avila P, Alvarez-Tejado M, Gutierrez MD, Garcia-Pardo A, Sanchez-Madrid F, et al. Role of the von Hippel-Lindau tumor suppressor gene in the formation of beta1-integrin fibrillar adhesions. Cancer Res. 2002;62(10):2929–36. Epub 2002/05/23.
66. Roe JS, Kim H, Lee SM, Kim ST, Cho EJ, Youn HD. p53 stabilization and transactivation by a von Hippel-Lindau protein. Mol Cell. 2006;22(3):395–405. Epub 2006/05/09.
67. Roe JS, Kim HR, Hwang IY, Ha NC, Kim ST, Cho EJ, et al. Phosphorylation of von Hippel–Lindau protein by checkpoint kinase 2 regulates p53 transactivation. Cell Cycle. 2011;10(22):3920–8. Epub 2011/11/11.
68. Yang H, Minamishima YA, Yan Q, Schlisio S, Ebert BL, Zhang X, et al. pVHL acts as an adaptor to promote the inhibitory phosphorylation of the NF-kappaB agonist Card9 by CK2. Mol Cell. 2007;28(1):15–27. Epub 2007/10/16.
69. Neurofibromatosis. Conference statement. National Institutes of Health Consensus Development Conference. Arch Neurol. 1988;45(5):575–8. Epub 1988/05/01.
70. Ferner RE, Huson SM, Thomas N, Moss C, Willshaw H, Evans DG, et al. Guidelines for the diagnosis and management of individuals with neurofibromatosis 1. J Med Genet. 2007;44(2):81–8. Epub 2006/11/16.
71. Garbrecht N, Anlauf M, Schmitt A, Henopp T, Sipos B, Raffel A, et al. Somatostatin-producing neuroendocrine tumors of the duodenum and pancreas: incidence, types, biological behavior, association with inherited syndromes, and functional activity. Endocr Relat Cancer. 2008;15(1):229–41. Epub 2008/03/04.
72. Patil S, Chamberlain RS. Neoplasms associated with germline and somatic NF1 gene mutations. Oncologist. 2012;17(1):101–16. Epub 2012/01/14.
73. Mao C, Shah A, Hanson DJ, Howard JM. Von Recklinghausen's disease associated with duodenal somatostatinoma: contrast of duodenal versus pancreatic somatostatinomas. J Surg Oncol. 1995;59(1):67–73. Epub 1995/05/01.
74. Usui M, Matsuda S, Suzuki H, Hirata K, Ogura Y, Shiraishi T. Somatostatinoma of the papilla of Vater with multiple gastrointestinal stromal tumors in a patient with von Recklinghausen's disease. J Gastroenterol. 2002;37(11):947–53. Epub 2002/12/17.
75. Le LQ, Parada LF. Tumor microenvironment and neurofibromatosis type I: connecting the GAPs. Oncogene. 2007;26(32):4609–16. Epub 2007/02/14.

76. Johannessen CM, Johnson BW, Williams SM, Chan AW, Reczek EE, Lynch RC, et al. TORC1 is essential for NF1-associated malignancies. Curr Biol. 2008;18(1):56–62. Epub 2008/01/01.
77. Johannessen CM, Reczek EE, James MF, Brems H, Legius E, Cichowski K. The NF1 tumor suppressor critically regulates TSC2 and mTOR. Proc Natl Acad Sci U S A. 2005; 102(24):8573–8. Epub 2005/06/07.
78. Northrup H, Krueger DA. Tuberous sclerosis complex diagnostic criteria update: recommendations of the 2012 international tuberous sclerosis complex consensus conference. Pediatr Neurol. 2013;49(4):243–54. Epub 2013/09/24.
79. Dabora SL, Jozwiak S, Franz DN, Roberts PS, Nieto A, Chung J, et al. Mutational analysis in a cohort of 224 tuberous sclerosis patients indicates increased severity of TSC2, compared with TSC1, disease in multiple organs. Am J Hum Genet. 2001;68(1):64–80. Epub 2000/12/12.
80. Sancak O, Nellist M, Goedbloed M, Elfferich P, Wouters C, Maat-Kievit A, et al. Mutational analysis of the TSC1 and TSC2 genes in a diagnostic setting: genotype–phenotype correlations and comparison of diagnostic DNA techniques in Tuberous Sclerosis Complex. Eur J Hum Genet. 2005;13(6):731–41. Epub 2005/03/31.
81. Au KS, Williams AT, Gambello MJ, Northrup H. Molecular genetic basis of tuberous sclerosis complex: from bench to bedside. J Child Neurol. 2004;19(9):699–709. Epub 2004/11/26.
82. Au KS, Williams AT, Roach ES, Batchelor L, Sparagana SP, Delgado MR, et al. Genotype/phenotype correlation in 325 individuals referred for a diagnosis of tuberous sclerosis complex in the United States. Genet Med. 2007;9(2):88–100. Epub 2007/02/17.
83. Maheshwar MM, Cheadle JP, Jones AC, Myring J, Fryer AE, Harris PC, et al. The GAP-related domain of tuberin, the product of the TSC2 gene, is a target for missense mutations in tuberous sclerosis. Hum Mol Genet. 1997;6(11):1991–6. Epub 1997/09/25.
84. Arva NC, Pappas JG, Bhatla T, Raetz EA, Macari M, Ginsburg HB, et al. Well-differentiated pancreatic neuroendocrine carcinoma in tuberous sclerosis–case report and review of the literature. Am J Surg Pathol. 2012;36(1):149–53. Epub 2011/12/17.
85. Fujimori M, Ikeda S, Shimizu Y, Okajima M, Asahara T. Accumulation of beta-catenin protein and mutations in exon 3 of beta-catenin gene in gastrointestinal carcinoid tumor. Cancer Res. 2001;61(18):6656–9. Epub 2001/09/18.
86. Perren A, Anlauf M, Komminoth P. Molecular profiles of gastroenteropancreatic endocrine tumors. Virchows Arch. 2007;451 Suppl 1:S39–46. Epub 2007/08/09.
87. Beghelli S, Pelosi G, Zamboni G, Falconi M, Iacono C, Bordi C, et al. Pancreatic endocrine tumours: evidence for a tumour suppressor pathogenesis and for a tumour suppressor gene on chromosome 17p. J Pathol. 1998;186(1):41–50. Epub 1999/01/06.
88. Jonkers YM, Claessen SM, Veltman JA, Geurts van Kessel A, Dinjens WN, Skogseid B, et al. Molecular parameters associated with insulinoma progression: chromosomal instability versus p53 and CK19 status. Cytogenet Genome Res. 2006;115(3–4):289–97. Epub 2006/11/25.
89. Moore PS, Orlandini S, Zamboni G, Capelli P, Rigaud G, Falconi M, et al. Pancreatic tumours: molecular pathways implicated in ductal cancer are involved in ampullary but not in exocrine nonductal or endocrine tumorigenesis. Br J Cancer. 2001;84(2):253–62. Epub 2001/02/13.
90. Perren A, Komminoth P, Saremaslani P, Matter C, Feurer S, Lees JA, et al. Mutation and expression analyses reveal differential subcellular compartmentalization of PTEN in endocrine pancreatic tumors compared to normal islet cells. Am J Pathol. 2000;157(4):1097–103. Epub 2000/10/06.
91. Serrano J, Goebel SU, Peghini PL, Lubensky IA, Gibril F, Jensen RT. Alterations in the p16INK4a/CDKN2A tumor suppressor gene in gastrinomas. J Clin Endocrinol Metab. 2000;85(11):4146–56. Epub 2000/11/30.
92. Yashiro T, Fulton N, Hara H, Yasuda K, Montag A, Yashiro N, et al. Comparison of mutations of ras oncogene in human pancreatic exocrine and endocrine tumors. Surgery. 1993; 114(4):758–63. discussion 63–4. Epub 1993/10/01.
93. Krausch M, Raffel A, Anlauf M, Schott M, Willenberg H, Lehwald N, et al. Loss of PTEN expression in neuroendocrine pancreatic tumors. Horm Metab Res. 2011;43(12):865–71. Epub 2011/11/23.

94. Muscarella P, Melvin WS, Fisher WE, Foor J, Ellison EC, Herman JG, et al. Genetic alterations in gastrinomas and nonfunctioning pancreatic neuroendocrine tumors: an analysis of p16/MTS1 tumor suppressor gene inactivation. Cancer Res. 1998;58(2):237–40. Epub 1998/01/27.
95. Komminoth P, Roth J, Muletta-Feurer S, Saremaslani P, Seelentag WK, Heitz PU. RET proto-oncogene point mutations in sporadic neuroendocrine tumors. J Clin Endocrinol Metab. 1996;81(6):2041–6. Epub 1996/06/01.
96. Perren A, Schmid S, Locher T, Saremaslani P, Bonvin C, Heitz PU, et al. BRAF and endocrine tumors: mutations are frequent in papillary thyroid carcinomas, rare in endocrine tumors of the gastrointestinal tract and not detected in other endocrine tumors. Endocr Relat Cancer. 2004;11(4):855–60. Epub 2004/12/23.
97. Shattuck TM, Costa J, Bernstein M, Jensen RT, Chung DC, Arnold A. Mutational analysis of Smad3, a candidate tumor suppressor implicated in TGF-beta and menin pathways, in parathyroid adenomas and enteropancreatic endocrine tumors. J Clin Endocrinol Metab. 2002;87(8):3911–4. Epub 2002/08/06.
98. Tannapfel A, Vomschloss S, Karhoff D, Markwarth A, Hengge UR, Wittekind C, et al. BRAF gene mutations are rare events in gastroenteropancreatic neuroendocrine tumors. Am J Clin Pathol. 2005;123(2):256–60. Epub 2005/04/22.
99. Bartsch D, Hahn SA, Danichevski KD, Ramaswamy A, Bastian D, Galehdari H, et al. Mutations of the DPC4/Smad4 gene in neuroendocrine pancreatic tumors. Oncogene. 1999;18(14):2367–71. Epub 1999/05/18.
100. Perren A, Saremaslani P, Schmid S, Bonvin C, Locher T, Roth J, et al. DPC4/Smad4: no mutations, rare allelic imbalances, and retained protein expression in pancreatic endocrine tumors. Diagn Mol Pathol. 2003;12(4):181–6. Epub 2003/11/26.
101. Lawrence MS, Stojanov P, Polak P, Kryukov GV, Cibulskis K, Sivachenko A, et al. Mutational heterogeneity in cancer and the search for new cancer-associated genes. Nature. 2013;499(7457):214–8. Epub 2013/06/19.
102. Yao JC, Shah MH, Ito T, Bohas CL, Wolin EM, Van Cutsem E, et al. Everolimus for advanced pancreatic neuroendocrine tumors. N Engl J Med. 2011;364(6):514–23. Epub 2011/02/11.
103. Yachida S, Vakiani E, White CM, Zhong Y, Saunders T, Morgan R, et al. Small cell and large cell neuroendocrine carcinomas of the pancreas are genetically similar and distinct from well-differentiated pancreatic neuroendocrine tumors. Am J Surg Pathol. 2012;36(2):173–84. Epub 2012/01/19.
104. Marinoni I, Kurrer AS, Vassella E, Dettmer M, Rudolph T, Banz V, et al. Loss of DAXX and ATRX are Associated with Chromosome Instability and Reduced Survival of Patients with Pancreatic Neuroendocrine Tumors. Gastroenterology. 2014;146(2):453–60. Epub 2013/10/24.
105. Gibbons RJ, Picketts DJ, Higgs DR. Syndromal mental retardation due to mutations in a regulator of gene expression. Hum Mol Genet. 1995;4:1705–9. Epub 1995/01/01.
106. De La Fuente R, Baumann C, Viveiros MM. Role of ATRX in chromatin structure and function: implications for chromosome instability and human disease. Reproduction. 2011;142(2):221–34. Epub 2011/06/10.
107. Law MJ, Lower KM, Voon HP, Hughes JR, Garrick D, Viprakasit V, et al. ATR-X syndrome protein targets tandem repeats and influences allele-specific expression in a size-dependent manner. Cell. 2010;143(3):367–78. Epub 2010/10/30.
108. Watson LA, Solomon LA, Li JR, Jiang Y, Edwards M, Shin-ya K, et al. Atrx deficiency induces telomere dysfunction, endocrine defects, and reduced life span. J Clin Invest. 2013;123(5):2049–63. Epub 2013/04/09.
109. Gibbons RJ, Wada T, Fisher CA, Malik N, Mitson MJ, Steensma DP, et al. Mutations in the chromatin-associated protein ATRX. Hum Mutat. 2008;29(6):796–802. Epub 2008/04/15.
110. Garrick D, Sharpe JA, Arkell R, Dobbie L, Smith AJ, Wood WG, et al. Loss of Atrx affects trophoblast development and the pattern of X-inactivation in extraembryonic tissues. PLoS Genet. 2006;2(4):e58. Epub 2006/04/22.
111. Dawson MA, Kouzarides T. Cancer epigenetics: from mechanism to therapy. Cell. 2012;150(1):12–27. Epub 2012/07/10.

112. Drane P, Ouararhni K, Depaux A, Shuaib M, Hamiche A. The death-associated protein DAXX is a novel histone chaperone involved in the replication-independent deposition of H3.3. Genes Dev. 2010;24(12):1253–65. Epub 2010/05/28.
113. Lewis PW, Elsaesser SJ, Noh KM, Stadler SC, Allis CD. Daxx is an H3.3-specific histone chaperone and cooperates with ATRX in replication-independent chromatin assembly at telomeres. Proc Natl Acad Sci U S A. 2010;107(32):14075–80.
114. Heaphy CM, de Wilde RF, Jiao Y, Klein AP, Edil BH, Shi C, et al. Altered telomeres in tumors with ATRX and DAXX mutations. Science. 2011;333(6041):425. Epub 2011/07/02.
115. de Wilde RF, Heaphy CM, Maitra A, Meeker AK, Edil BH, Wolfgang CL, et al. Loss of ATRX or DAXX expression and concomitant acquisition of the alternative lengthening of telomeres phenotype are late events in a small subset of MEN-1 syndrome pancreatic neuroendocrine tumors. Mod Pathol. 2012;25(7):1033–9. Epub 2012/05/12.
116. Heaphy CM, Subhawong AP, Hong SM, Goggins MG, Montgomery EA, Gabrielson E, et al. Prevalence of the alternative lengthening of telomeres telomere maintenance mechanism in human cancer subtypes. Am J Pathol. 2011;179(4):1608–15. Epub 2011/09/06.
117. Maitra A, Hansel DE, Argani P, Ashfaq R, Rahman A, Naji A, et al. Global expression analysis of well-differentiated pancreatic endocrine neoplasms using oligonucleotide microarrays. Clin Cancer Res. 2003;9(16 Pt 1):5988–95. Epub 2003/12/17.
118. Hansel DE, Rahman A, House M, Ashfaq R, Berg K, Yeo CJ, et al. Met proto-oncogene and insulin-like growth factor binding protein 3 overexpression correlates with metastatic ability in well-differentiated pancreatic endocrine neoplasms. Clin Cancer Res. 2004;10(18 Pt 1): 6152–8. Epub 2004/09/28.
119. Couvelard A, Hu J, Steers G, O'Toole D, Sauvanet A, Belghiti J, et al. Identification of potential therapeutic targets by gene-expression profiling in pancreatic endocrine tumors. Gastroenterology. 2006;131(5):1597–610. Epub 2006/10/27.
120. Capurso G, Lattimore S, Crnogorac-Jurcevic T, Panzuto F, Milione M, Bhakta V, et al. Gene expression profiles of progressive pancreatic endocrine tumours and their liver metastases reveal potential novel markers and therapeutic targets. Endocr Relat Cancer. 2006;13(2):541–58. Epub 2006/05/27.
121. Bloomston M, Durkin A, Yang I, Rojiani M, Rosemurgy AS, Enkmann S, et al. Identification of molecular markers specific for pancreatic neuroendocrine tumors by genetic profiling of core biopsies. Ann Surg Oncol. 2004;11(4):413–9. Epub 2004/04/09.
122. Missiaglia E, Dalai I, Barbi S, Beghelli S, Falconi M, Dellaperuta M, et al. Pancreatic endocrine tumors: expression profiling evidences a role for AKT-mTOR pathway. J Clin Oncol. 2010;28(2):245–55. Epub 2009/11/18.
123. Nasir A, Helm J, Turner L, Chen DT, Strosberg J, Hafez N, et al. RUNX1T1: a novel predictor of liver metastasis in primary pancreatic endocrine neoplasms. Pancreas. 2011;40(4):627–33. Epub 2011/04/19.
124. Speel EJ, Scheidweiler AF, Zhao J, Matter C, Saremaslani P, Roth J, et al. Genetic evidence for early divergence of small functioning and nonfunctioning endocrine pancreatic tumors: gain of 9Q34 is an early event in insulinomas. Cancer Res. 2001;61(13):5186–92. Epub 2001/06/30.
125. Zhao J, Moch H, Scheidweiler AF, Baer A, Schaffer AA, Speel EJ, et al. Genomic imbalances in the progression of endocrine pancreatic tumors. Genes Chromosomes Cancer. 2001; 32(4):364–72. Epub 2001/12/18.
126. Stumpf E, Aalto Y, Hoog A, Kjellman M, Otonkoski T, Knuutila S, et al. Chromosomal alterations in human pancreatic endocrine tumors. Genes Chromosomes Cancer. 2000; 29(1):83–7. Epub 2000/08/05.
127. Speel EJ, Richter J, Moch H, Egenter C, Saremaslani P, Rutimann K, et al. Genetic differences in endocrine pancreatic tumor subtypes detected by comparative genomic hybridization. Am J Pathol. 1999;155(6):1787–94. Epub 1999/12/14.
128. Dammann R, Schagdarsurengin U, Liu L, Otto N, Gimm O, Dralle H, et al. Frequent RASSF1A promoter hypermethylation and K-ras mutations in pancreatic carcinoma. Oncogene. 2003;22(24):3806–12. Epub 2003/06/13.

129. House MG, Herman JG, Guo MZ, Hooker CM, Schulick RD, Lillemoe KD, et al. Aberrant hypermethylation of tumor suppressor genes in pancreatic endocrine neoplasms. Ann Surg. 2003;238(3):423–31. discussion 31-2. Epub 2003/09/23.
130. Malpeli G, Amato E, Dandrea M, Fumagalli C, Debattisti V, Boninsegna L, et al. Methylation-associated down-regulation of RASSF1A and up-regulation of RASSF1C in pancreatic endocrine tumors. BMC Cancer. 2011;11:351. Epub 2011/08/16.
131. Pizzi S, Azzoni C, Bottarelli L, Campanini N, D'Adda T, Pasquali C, et al. RASSF1A promoter methylation and 3p21.3 loss of heterozygosity are features of foregut, but not midgut and hindgut, malignant endocrine tumours. J Pathol. 2005;206(4):409–16.
132. Bartsch DK, Kersting M, Wild A, Ramaswamy A, Gerdes B, Schuermann M, et al. Low frequency of p16(INK4a) alterations in insulinomas. Digestion. 2000;62(2–3):171–7. Epub 2000/10/12.
133. Chan AO, Kim SG, Bedeir A, Issa JP, Hamilton SR, Rashid A. CpG island methylation in carcinoid and pancreatic endocrine tumors. Oncogene. 2003;22(6):924–34. Epub 2003/02/14.
134. Wild A, Ramaswamy A, Langer P, Celik I, Fendrich V, Chaloupka B, et al. Frequent methylation-associated silencing of the tissue inhibitor of metalloproteinase-3 gene in pancreatic endocrine tumors. J Clin Endocrinol Metab. 2003;88(3):1367–73. Epub 2003/03/12.
135. Arnold CN, Sosnowski A, Schmitt-Graff A, Arnold R, Blum HE. Analysis of molecular pathways in sporadic neuroendocrine tumors of the gastro-entero-pancreatic system. Int J Cancer. 2007;120(10):2157–64. Epub 2007/02/06.
136. Banck MS, Kanwar R, Kulkarni AA, Boora GK, Metge F, Kipp BR, et al. The genomic landscape of small intestine neuroendocrine tumors. J Clin Invest. 2013;123(6):2502–8. Epub 2013/05/17.
137. Zikusoka MN, Kidd M, Eick G, Latich I, Modlin IM. The molecular genetics of gastroentero-pancreatic neuroendocrine tumors. Cancer. 2005;104(11):2292–309. Epub 2005/11/01.
138. Kulke MH, Freed E, Chiang DY, Philips J, Zahrieh D, Glickman JN, et al. High-resolution analysis of genetic alterations in small bowel carcinoid tumors reveals areas of recurrent amplification and loss. Genes Chromosomes Cancer. 2008;47(7):591–603. Epub 2008/04/03.

Chapter 3
Laboratory Assessment of NETs

Christos Toumpanakis

3.1 Introduction

Pancreatic neuroendocrine tumors (pNETs) are derived from the endocrine cells of the pancreatic islets of Langerhans and may be *functioning or non-functioning*. In the former group, the predominant symptoms are those of the hormonal hypersecretion. These tumors get their name from the predominant peptide that they secrete. The most common ones include gastrinomas, insulinomas, vaso-active intestinal polypeptide (VIP)-omas, glucagonomas, somatostatinomas, growth-hormone releasing factor secreting tumors (GRF-omas), and ACTH secreting tumors of the pancreas (ACTH-omas). Other rarer pNETs have recently been considered as causing syndromes, including pNETs causing hypercalcemia [producing parathormone (PTH) and parathormone-related peptide (PTH-rp)], pNETs secreting calcitonin, and finally serotonin producing pNETs. In non-functioning tumors, symptoms are associated to the mechanical effects of tumor mass itself. However, non-functioning pNETs may produce hormones as well, but remain clinically silent for the following reasons: (a) the hormones produced may not develop a known specific clinical syndrome [pancreatic polypeptide (PP) omas], (b) the tumor may produce a known peptide, but fails to release it, or (c) the tumor produces biologically inactive precursor forms of hormones [1].

The diagnosis of pNETs is based upon: (a) the clinical features, especially in functioning tumors, (b) the levels of several peptides and amines, that represent tumor products, in blood and urine (biomarkers), (c) the localization of primary and/or metastatic lesions by imaging studies, and (d) the histopathological confirmation (through a biopsy or a surgical specimen) which represents the "gold standard" and should be obtained whenever possible.

C. Toumpanakis, M.D., Ph.D. (✉)
Centre for Gastroenterology, Neuroendocrine Tumour Unit,
Royal Free Hospital, London NW3 2QG, UK
e-mail: c.toumpanakis@ucl.ac.uk

J.R. Pisegna (ed.), *Management of Pancreatic Neuroendocrine Tumors*,
DOI 10.1007/978-1-4939-1798-3_3

Clinical features that may raise the suspicion for gastrinoma include recurrent and resistant to treatment peptic ulcers, which are not related to *Helicobacter pylori* or non-steroidal anti-inflammatory drugs (NSAIDs), erosive oesophagitis and chronic diarrhea, associated to hypergastrinaemia; patients with insulinomas develop symptoms (e.g., faintness, perspiration) as a result of hypoglycemia, secondary to insulin hypersecretion; VIPomas patients have a severe secretory diarrhea, which causes dehydration and hypokalaemia, due to VIP hypersecretion. Additionally, in patients with glucagonomas, a characteristic necrolytic migratory erythema, in combination with weight loss and diabetes mellitus, may occur as systemic effects of glucagon hypersecretion [2].

In this chapter, we are focusing on the laboratory assessment of pNETs and will present all established and novel *biomarkers* that are used: (a) to confirm a clinically suspected hormonal syndrome or a non-functioning pNET that was revealed incidentally by imaging studies, (b) in follow-up assessments and surveillance for disease recurrence after a surgical treatment, (c) for prediction and monitoring of treatment response, and (d) for prognostic purposes.

3.2 Biomarkers

Biomarkers are cellular (histological), biochemical, and molecular (including genetic) substances that can be objectively measured in biological media, such as tissue or fluids. Neuroendocrine cells can produce and secrete several peptides and biogenic amines that can be measured in serum and urine and may serve as biomarkers. Some of these markers may be *specific* for a clinical syndrome associated with these tumors, whereas others are thought to be *non-specific (general)*, as they are secreted by a variety of neuroendocrine cells [3].

3.2.1 Specific

Specific biomarkers for the most common functioning pNETs include the following hormonal peptides: gastrin (gastrinoma), insulin, C-peptide, and proinsulin (insulinoma), glucagon (glucagonoma), VIP (VIPoma), and somatostatin (somatostatinoma). As most of these substances represent gut hormones, they should be assessed after, at least, 6-h fast. Relevant symptoms associated with raised levels of the above-noted peptides strongly indicate the presence of a functioning pNET. However, in some of these tumors, raised hormonal levels alone are not enough to establish the diagnosis.

The biochemical confirmation, following a clinical suspicion, of a gastrinoma requires a significant elevation of *fasting serum gastrin*, in combination with hypechlorhydria. The presence of the latter is very important, as hypergastrinemia alone can be result of chronic hypochlorhydria/achlorhydria, that is associated with chronic fundus atrophic gastritis, chronic proton pump inhibitors' (PPIs) use, as well as vagotomy [4].

Table 3.1 Differential diagnosis of hypergastrinaemia

	Gastric p H<2	Gastric p H>2
Gastrin levels >10-folds of the upper normal limit	*Diagnosis of gastrinoma*	*Consider other causes* (atrophic gastritis, chronic PPI use, vagotomy)
Gastrin levels <10-folds of the upper normal limit	*First exclude other causes* *H. pylori* infection, gastric outlet obstruction, antral G cell hyperplasia, short bowel syndrome, retained antrum or renal failure *And then* perform "Secretin Test"	*Consider other causes* (atrophic gastritis, chronic PPI use, vagotomy)

A fasting serum gastrin (*gastin-17*) *level* of >10-fold the upper normal limit, in the presence of gastric pH<2 or basic acid output (BAO)>15 mmol/h, is considered as diagnostic of a gastrinoma. If possible, PPIs should be discontinued at least 10 days, prior to serum gastrin estimation, while a discontinuation of Histamine-2 receptor (H2R) antagonists for only 48–72 h prior to the test seems to be adequate. Moderately elevated serum gastrin levels (<10-fold the upper normal limit) and hypechlorhydria may occur in 66 % of gastrinoma patients, but in this scenario other clinical entities can be also considered, such as *H. pylori* infection, gastric outlet obstruction, antral G cell hyperplasia, short bowel syndrome, retained antrum, or renal failure. For differential diagnosis, a provocative test with intravenous (IV) administration of secretin is performed, as follows: after an overnight fast an IV bolus of secretin (2 U/kg) is given to the patient. A rise of serum gastrin concentration >120 pg/mL, noted within 10 min of secretin administration, can establish the diagnosis of gastrinoma, whereas in the above-mentioned non-gastrinoma-related causes, serum gastrin levels remain practically unchanged. It has been recently recommended that PPIs need also to be discontinued, prior to the secretin provocative test [5]. The differential diagnosis of hypergastrinaemia is summarized in Table 3.1.

Similarly, whenever insulinoma is clinically suspected, the following six criteria are required in order to confirm the biochemical diagnosis: (1) blood glucose levels 2.2 mmol/L (40 mg/dL) or less, (2) concomitant insulin levels 6 μU/mL or greater, (3) C-peptide levels 200 pmol/L or greater, (4) proinsulin levels 5 pmol/L or greater, (5) β-hydroxybutyrate levels 2.7 mmol/L or less, and (6) absence of sulfonylurea metabolites in plasma and urine. If diagnosis is still unclear, a 72 h fast test is performed into the hospital. When the patient develops hypoglycaemic symptoms and blood glucose is low, plasma insulin, proinsulin, and C-peptide levels are measured. Low blood glucose levels, associated with inappropriately high plasma insulin, proinsulin, and C-peptide levels, at the same time strongly indicate the autonomous secretion of insulin [6].

In a patient with radiologically ± histologically proven pNET, rare clinical entities should be suspected if: (a) hypecalcaemia with normal PTH levels is noted. This may indicate a PTH-rp secreting tumor, and PTH-rp needs to be measured; and (b) symptoms of carcinoid syndrome (flushing, diarrhea, bronchospasm) are reported. In this scenario, a serotonin-producing functioning pNET may be present and therefore urinary 5-hydroxyindoleacetic acid (5-HIAA), a breakdown product of serotonin, needs to be measured in a 24-h urine collection. During this collection, the patients should be avoiding certain foods like bananas, avocados, aubergine, pineapples, plums, walnuts, and some drugs like paracetamol, fluorouracil, methysergide, naproxen, and caffeine, which may cause false positive results. On the contrary, other drugs like levodopa or phenothiazines may result in false negative results.

3.2.2 Non-specific (General)

3.2.2.1 Chromogranin-A (CgA)

Chromogranins are a family of water-soluble acidic glycoproteins, including at least three different members (CgA, CgB, CgC), which are stored in the secretory granules of neuroendocrine cells and released during exocytosis. Plasma CgA is found throughout the diffuse neuroendocrine system and is thought to be the best and most sensitive general marker for the diagnosis and follow-up of gastro-entero-pancreatic NETs. Its plasma levels may correlate with tumor progression or regression and also their alteration may precede radiographic evidence of progression. The sensitivity of plasma CgA is 96 % and 75 % in functioning and non-functioning pNETs, respectively, while its specificity varies from 68 to 100 % [7]. The sensitivity and specificity of circulating CgA in clinical practice depends on several factors including tumor type and tumor volume. For example, benign insulinomas and small volume tumors may have normal circulating levels of CgA, which results in false negative results. Also, poorly differentiated endocrine carcinomas usually have low CgA expression and therefore are associated with low or normal circulating CgA levels [8]. On the contrary, CgA may be raised in several non-neoplastic clinical entities such as atrophic gastritis, chronic use of PPIs, renal failure, hepatic failure, inflammatory bowel disease, etc. and some non-NET malignancies such as breast cancer, prostate cancer, ovarian cancer, colorectal cancer, hepatocellular carcinoma, etc. [9]. Therefore, the presence of any of the above-noted situations needs to be taken into account when interpreting CgA levels. Finally, apart from benign insulinomas, its clinical value is limited in patients with gastrinomas. In those patients, there is not precise correlation of tumor burden with CgA levels, as CgA may also be produced by the enterochromaffin-like cells of stomach in response to hypergastrinemia [10]. On the basis of the above, it is reasonable to interpret CgA levels, especially in pNETs, in combination with the specific tumor markers associated with them (i.e., gastrin in gastrinomas, VIP in VIPomas, etc.). Finally, although in midgut NETs, significantly raised CgA at diagnosis is associated with worse survival, the role of this markers as a prognostic factor has not been well established in pNETs so far.

3.2.2.2 Other Members of Chromogranin Family

Pancreastatin is a breakdown product of CgA resulting from the action of prohormone convertase-1. Pancreastatin is considered more sensitive than CgA and may be used to identify NETs with small tumor volumes or the early stages of development of liver metastases, when CgA levels may still be normal. Pancreastatin may thus be useful in diagnosing NETs at a very early stage or in detecting early recurrence. Of note, assays measuring the middle of the pancreastatin molecule cross-react with CgA, while those measuring the C- and N-terminals of pancreastatin do not. These C- and N-terminal assays may be of clinical utility as pancreastatin is not raised in gastric achlorhydria. Therefore, false positives may occur less frequently with pancreastatin than CgA in certain patient groups [11]. However, pancreastatin is not widely available.

CgB (also known as secretogranin I) is a less sensitive biomarker than CgA. The exceptions include MEN-1-related tumors and benign insulinomas, where CgA levels may be within normal limits [12]. Circulating CgC (secretogranin II) currently has no formal role in the follow-up and treatment of NETs.

3.2.2.3 Pancreatic Polypeptide

PP is produced by normal pancreatic islet cells. Its circulating levels can be raised in approximately 80 % of pNETs. Its sensitivity is reportedly lower than that of CgA. However, when used in combination with CgA, sensitivity increases to 95 % for pNETs. PP has low specificity, however, as it may be also raised in patients with diarrhea due to other causes and in patients with diabetes [13].

3.2.2.4 Neuron-Specific Enolase

Neuron-specific enolase (NSE) is an isomer of a glycolytic enzyme found in neurons and neuroendocrine cells, and may also serve as a circulating non-specific marker for NETs. NSE is more frequently raised in patients with small cell lung carcinomas (74 %), and also medullary thyroid carcinomas and pheochromocytomas. Its sensitivity in NETs is rather low (40 %) and also its specificity is lower than plasma CgA. However, circulating NSE levels seem to have greater clinical utility than CgA in poorly differentiated neuroendocrine carcinomas, as these tumors often express NSE [14].

3.2.2.5 Common Tumor Markers

From the tumor markers that are used in other common cancers, alpha-Fetoprotein (a-FP) can be raised in some NETs and it may be possible to use AFP levels to identify subsets of patients with aggressive NET and therefore unfavorable prognosis [15].

3.3 Novel Biomarkers

Circulating tumor cells (CTCs) are a novel NET biomarker currently under evaluation. Previous research in other solid tumors, using the CellSearch® (Veridex) platform, has enabled quantification and characterization of CTCs in breast, colorectal, and prostate cancer. It has been demonstrated that the majority of NETs express the epithelial cell adhesion molecule and CTCs can therefore be detected using the

CellSearch platform in NET patients. Recent data in patients with metastatic NETs have demonstrated that the presence of CTCs was a significant prognostic marker for progression free and overall survival, based on multivariate analysis [16].

3.3.1 Other Laboratory Tests

3.3.1.1 Serum Calcium and Parathyroid Hormone Levels

Serum calcium and parathyroid hormone (PTH) levels should be requested as screening tests for MEN-1 syndrome in every patient with pNET at the time of diagnosis, as this association may have significant implications in patients' management and prognosis. Also, once MEN-1 diagnosis is established in an index case, a MEN-1 germline mutation DNA test should be performed in all his kindred after their first decade of life, and MEN-1 mutation carriers should be in a surveillance program [17].

In Fig. 3.1 and Table 3.2, we summarize the laboratory assessment of pNETs at diagnosis and follow-up, respectively.

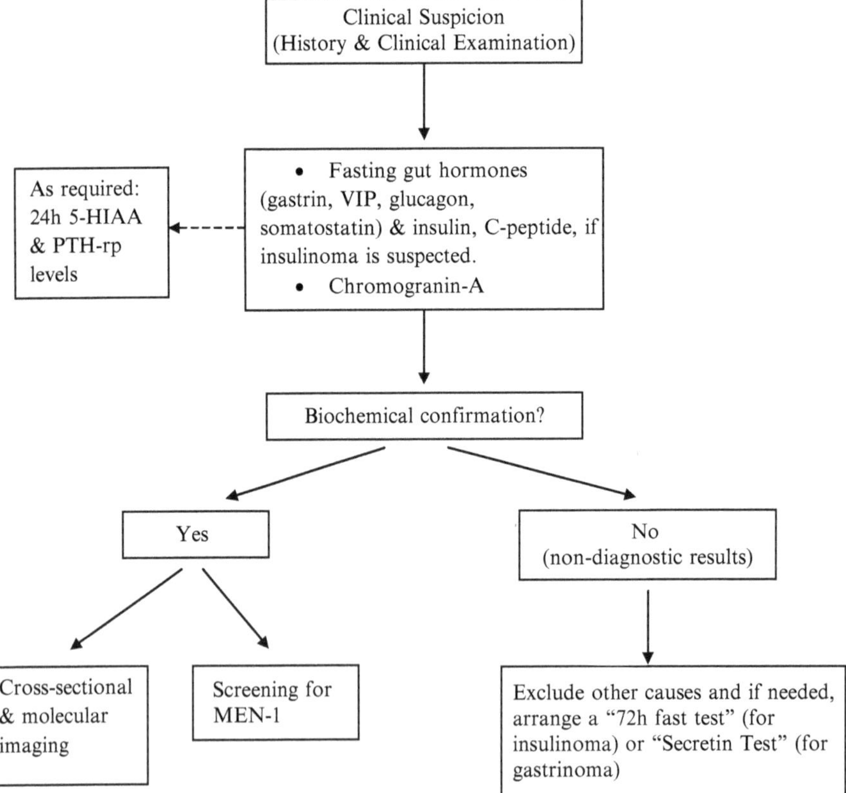

Fig. 3.1 Initial laboratory assessment of patients with clinically suspected pNET. *Note*: If the tumor has already been proven, the laboratory assessment at diagnosis includes (a) Fasting gut hormones (b) Chromogranin-A, and (c) screening for MEN-1

Table 3.2 Suggested laboratory investigations for follow-up of pNETs

	Functioning	Non-Functioning
Well-differentiated NETs	• Fasting gut hormones or Insulin • Chromogranin-A	• Chromogranin-A
Poorly differentiated NEC (neuroendocrine carcinomas)	• Fasting gut hormones or Insulin • Chromogranin-A • (NSE) • (a-FP)	• Chromogranin-A • (NSE) • (a-FP)

References

1. Oberg K. Pancreatic endocrine tumors. Semin Oncol. 2010;37:594–618.
2. Ekeblad S. Islet cell tumours. Adv Exp Med Biol. 2010;654:771–89.
3. Ardill JE, Erikkson B. The importance of the measurement of circulating markers in patients with neuroendocrine tumours of the pancreas and gut. Endocr Relat Cancer. 2003;10:459–62.
4. Caplin ME. Zollinger-Ellison syndrome. In: Modlin I, editor. From Gastrin to GERD a century of acid suppression. Hannover: Felsenstein; 2006.
5. Jensen RT. Gastrinomas: advances in diagnosis and management. Neuroendocrinology. 2004;80 Suppl 1:23–7.
6. Vanderveen K, Grant C. Insulinoma. Cancer Treat Res. 2010;153:235–52.
7. Arnold R, Wilke A, Rinke A, et al. Plasma chromogranin a as marker for survival in patients with metastatic endocrine gastroenteropancreatic tumors. Clin Gastroenterol Hepatol. 2008;6:820–7.
8. Lawrence B, Gustafsson BI, Kidd M, et al. The clinical relevance of chromogranin a as a biomarker for gastroenteropancreatic neuroendocrine tumors. Endocrinol Metab Clin North Am. 2011;40:111–34. viii.
9. Modlin IM, Gustafsson BI, Moss SF, et al. Chromogranin a—biological function and clinical utility in neuro endocrine tumor disease. Ann Surg Oncol. 2010;17:2427–43.
10. Campana D, Nori F, Piscitelli L, et al. Chromogranin A: is it a useful marker of neuroendocrine tumors? J Clin Oncol. 2007;25(15):1967–73.
11. O'Dorisio TM, Krutzik SR, Woltering EA, et al. Development of a highly sensitive and specific carboxy-terminal human pancreastatin assay to monitor neuroendocrine tumor behavior. Pancreas. 2010;39:611–6.
12. Ardill JE, O'Dorisio TM. Circulating biomarkers in neuroendocrine tumors of the enteropancreatic tract: Application to diagnosis, monitoring disease, and as prognostic indicators. Endocrinol Metab Clin North Am. 2010;39:777–90.
13. Oberg K. Neuroendocrine tumors of the gastrointestinal tract: recent advances in molecular genetics, diagnosis, and treatment. Curr Opin Oncol. 2005;17:386–91.
14. Berretta M, Cappellani A, Di Vita M, et al. Biomarkers in neuroendocrine tumors. Front Biosci (Schol Ed). 2010;2:332–42.
15. Shah T, Srirajaskanthan R, Bhogal M, et al. Alpha-fetoprotein and human chorionic gonadotrophin-beta as prognostic markers in neuroendocrine tumour patients. Br J Cancer. 2008;99:72–7.
16. Khan MS, Kirkwood A, Tsigani T, et al. Circulating tumor cells as prognostic markers in neuroendocrine tumors. J Clin Oncol. 2013;31:365–72.
17. Toumpanakis CG, Caplin ME. Molecular genetics of gastroenteropancreatic neuroendocrine tumors. Am J Gastroenterol. 2008;103(3):729–32.

Chapter 4
Zollinger–Ellison Syndrome: Diagnosis and Management

Maneesh H. Singh and David C. Metz

Abbreviations

BAO	Basal acid output
CT	Computed tomography
EGD	Esophagogastroduodenoscopy
FSG	Fasting serum gastrin
GERD	Gastroesophageal reflux disease
H2-R	H2-Receptor
MAO	Maximal acid output
MEN-1	Multiple endocrine neoplasia type 1
PET	Positron emission tomography
PPI	Proton-pump inhibitor
PRRT	Peptide receptor radionuclide therapy
PUD	Peptic ulcer disease
SRS	Somatostatin receptor scintigraphy
SST	Secretin stimulation testing
ZES	Zollinger–Ellison syndrome

M.H. Singh, M.D.
Department of Internal Medicine, Division of Gastroenterology, University of California, San Francisco, 513 Parnassus Avenue, Room S-357, San Francisco, CA 94143, USA

D.C. Metz, M.D. (✉)
Department of Internal Medicine, Perelman School of Medicine at the University of Pennsylvania, 9th floor Penn Tower, 1 Convention Ave, Philadelphia, PA 19104, USA

Division of Gastroenterology, Perelman School of Medicine at the University of Pennsylvania, 9th floor Penn Tower, 1 Convention Ave, Philadelphia, PA 19104, USA
e-mail: David.Metz@uphs.upenn.edu

J.R. Pisegna (ed.), *Management of Pancreatic Neuroendocrine Tumors*,
DOI 10.1007/978-1-4939-1798-3_4

4.1 Introduction

Over half a century has passed since Zollinger and Ellison first identified their eponymous triad of a non-beta islet cell tumor of the pancreas, gastric acid hypersecretion, and fulminant peptic ulcer disease (PUD) [1]. Since then, diagnostic and therapeutic strategies have advanced considerably; however, the proper workup and management of Zollinger–Ellison syndrome (ZES) still enlivens debate.

ZES is a rare clinical entity (1–3 cases/million/year diagnosed annually) characterized by gastric acid hypersecretion due to the exogenous release of gastrin by a neuroendocrine tumor usually found within the duodenum or pancreas. In about one-quarter to one-third of these patients [2–4], the tumor is associated with the presence of the multiple endocrine neoplasia type 1 (MEN-1) syndrome, while the remaining tumors are sporadic in origin. Older studies have shown about 60–90 % of these tumors to be malignant [5, 6], while a more recent study has found a subgroup of approximately 25 % to follow a particularly malignant course characterized by the development of liver metastases and significant morbidity and mortality [7]. Thus, prompt diagnosis and treatment of these patients is paramount. In this chapter, we discuss the clinical presentation of ZES, diagnostic strategies, the medical and surgical management of sporadic and MEN-1-associated cases, and the evolving landscape of advanced therapies for unresectable metastatic disease.

4.2 Clinical Presentation

Although many patients with ZES still present with the prototypical scenario of severe and complicated PUD (up to 5 % of patients still present with perforation [8]), this classical presentation actually represents only a minority of cases. In fact, the vast majority of ZES patients are virtually indistinguishable from the far more prevalent (>2300 cases/million/year) idiopathic PUD (Table 4.1). The presence of heartburn is similarly unhelpful as gastroesophageal reflux disease (GERD) is present to some degree in approximately 20 % of the US population [9]. With the advent of proton-pump inhibitor (PPI) therapy, many such patients are treated empirically early in their disease course and their actual diagnosis may remain masked. This has contributed to a delay in diagnosis of approximately 4–7 years after the initial onset of symptoms; a delay that has persisted for over four decades despite a general familiarity with ZES among physicians [4, 5, 10–12].

Given the overlap in symptomatology between ZES and other upper gastrointestinal disorders, a high index of suspicion is required for a timely diagnosis. Much of our current data on its clinical presentation is derived from several large prospective studies, in which ZES patients most commonly presented with symptoms of abdominal pain (75 %) and diarrhea (35–73 %; isolated in up to 35 %) though up to 60 % have coexisting acid reflux [4, 12–15]. Of course, abdominal pain and heartburn are

Table 4.1 Clinical features of patients with ZES and PUD (review of the literature)

	Zollinger–Ellison syndrome		Peptic ulcer disease	
Clinical feature	Mean	Range	Mean	95 % CI
Male	56	44–70	54	–
Age at onset, years	41	41–53	–	–
Duration of symptoms, years	5.2	3.2–8.7	–	–
Presenting symptom				
Abdominal pain	75 %	26–100 %	81 %	77–85 %
Diarrhea	73 %	35–73 %	–	–
Pain and diarrhea	55 %	28–60 %	–	–
Heartburn	44 %	0–64 %	46 %	42–50 %
Duodenal ulcers	71 %	71–93 %	–	–
Ulcer complications				
GI bleeding	24 %	8–75 %	29 %	25–34 %
Perforation	5 %	0–5 %	–	–
Obstruction	ND	0–5 %	–	–
With MEN-1	22 %	22–24 %	–	–

Data from Soga and Yakuwa (1998), Roy et al. (2000), Jensen (1998), Miller et al. (1990), Kaplan et al. (1990), Farley et al. (1992), Mignon and Cadiot (1998), Barkun and Leontiadis (2010), Schubert et al. (1993), Dent et al. (2010)

the defining symptoms of idiopathic PUD and GERD, respectively, such that these symptoms lack discriminant utility. Therefore, diagnosis requires the identification of a constellation of symptoms, clinical history, and radiographic signs which are summarized in Table 4.2. For example, diarrhea in association with other upper GI symptoms is a clinically distinctive feature distinguishing ZES patients from patients with idiopathic acid-peptic disease. This diarrhea is typically responsive to the addition or dose increase of PPI therapy or nasogastric aspiration suggesting gastric acid hypersecretion, a pathognomonic finding for ZES.

With esophagogastroduodenoscopy (EGD) being commonly performed in dyspeptic patients, endoscopic features may also play a role in diagnosis. Prominent gastric folds have been identified as a hallmark of the disease, reportedly found in approximately 94 % of patients with ZES in one large prospective study [4]. In addition, PUD in unusual locations (e.g., post-bulbar) and PUD in the absence of either *Helicobacter pylori* infection (only 10–50 % of ZES patients) or NSAID exposure should suggest the diagnosis of ZES [4, 16]. As mentioned earlier, MEN-1 is the cause of ZES in approximately one-quarter to one-third of patients; therefore, a personal or family history of extensive PUD or endocrinopathies (hyperparathyroidism, pancreatic endocrine tumors, carcinoids, and pituitary tumors) should prompt further investigation [2–4, 17].

As was alluded to earlier, the ubiquitous use of PPIs has complicated the diagnosis of ZES. Corleto et al. [18] investigated referral patterns at two well-known centers

Table 4.2 Clinical manifestations suggestive of ZES

Peptic ulcer disease or GERD…
With diarrhea
With weight loss
With long-standing, persistent symptoms refractory to treatment
With complication (bleeding, perforation, penetration)
Without *Helicobacter pylori* or NSAID-use
With endocrinopathy
Persistent diarrhea…
With abdominal pain
With esophageal disease/symptoms
With weight loss
Refractory to disease-specific treatment
Responsive to PPI therapy or secretory in nature
Endoscopic/Radiographic signs
Prominent gastric folds on endoscopy or upper GI series
Type 2 carcinoids (in MEN-1 syndrome)
Multiple peptic ulcers or ulcers in unusual locations (i.e., beyond duodenal bulb)
Esophageal stricture secondary to PUD
Family history…
Of peptic ulcer disease
Of hypercalcemia or nephrolithiasis due to primary hyperparathyroidism
Of hypoglycemia due to insulinoma
Of functioning or nonfunctioning pituitary tumor
Of diarrhea due to VIPoma

(the National Institutes of Health, Bethesda, MD and Universitá La Sapienza II, Rome, Italy) and reported that with the widespread adoption of PPIs, fewer patients are being referred for work-up of a possible gastrinoma diagnosis and fewer new patients are diagnosed annually. Specifically, they noted a 62 % decrease in referrals ($p<0.00001$) and a 40 % decrease in new case diagnoses ($p=0.002$) despite an increase in referrals of patients with other gastrointestinal pancreatic endocrine tumors (Fig. 4.1). Prior to PPIs, ZES patients were often found refractory to conventional doses of histamine H2-receptor (H2-R) antagonists used to treat idiopathic PUD or GERD, and also developed tachyphylaxis to higher doses offering clinicians a clue to the underlying diagnosis. PPIs at standard dosing, on the other hand, effectively control symptoms of idiopathic acid-peptic disease as well as the gastric acid hypersecretion associated with ZES in many patients, thereby masking the indication for additional work-up until symptoms progress, often with the onset of metastatic disease.

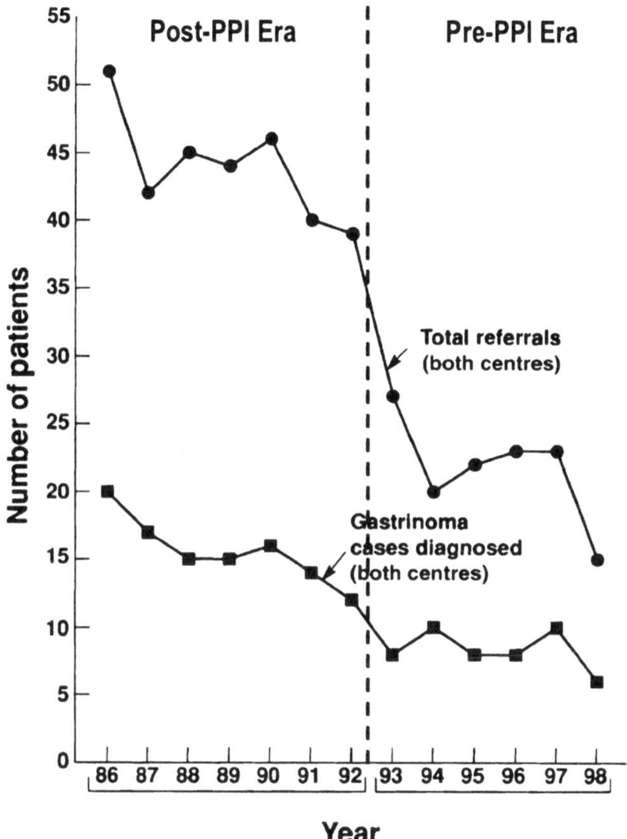

Fig. 4.1 *Effect of widespread PPI use on diagnosis and referral for diagnosis of ZES.* The number of referrals and diagnoses of new cases of ZES at the National Institutes of Health (Bethesda, MD) and Universitá La Sapienza II (Rome, Italy) in the pre- and post-PPI era. Both the annual number of referrals ($p=0.0020$) and the annual number of new diagnoses of ZES ($p=0.0006$) showed a significant decrease after the widespread use of PPIs. *Reproduced with permission from John Wiley and Sons, Corleto et al. (2001)*

4.3 Diagnosis

4.3.1 Hypergastrinemia

Gastrinomas secrete gastrin, a peptide hormone responsible for gastric acid hypersecretion. Hypergastrinemia may be the hallmark of ZES; however, diagnosis also requires demonstration of concomitant acid hypersecretion or, in other words, *inappropriate* hypergastrinemia. This entails an assessment of gastric acid secretory capability by gastric pH or basal acid output (BAO) measurement together with a fasting serum gastrin (FSG) level. The causes of hypergastrinemia are listed in Table 4.3

Table 4.3 Causes of hypergastrinemia

Causes of hypergastrinemia
Appropriate hypergastrinemia (elevated gastric pH)
Atrophic gastritis with or without pernicious anemia
Chronic proton pump inhibitor or H2-R antagonist therapy
Helicobacter pylori pangastritis
Post-vagotomy
Inappropriate hypergastrinemia (acidic gastric pH)
Gastrinoma (sporadic ZES or associated MEN-1)
Antral-predominant *Helicobacter pylori* gastritis
Gastric-outlet obstruction
Renal failure and uremia
Retained-antrum syndrome
Small-bowel resection
Spurious hypergastrinemia
Nonfasting patient
Inaccurate assay

Adapted from Metz (2012)

and are subdivided into two major categories based on gastric pH measurement: appropriate (with an elevated gastric pH) and inappropriate hypergastrinemia (with an acidic gastric pH) [19, 20]. A third category of hypergastrinemia, spurious hypergastrinemia, also needs to be considered (Table 4.3). Appropriate hypergastrinemia implies a physiologically appropriate increase in serum gastrin in response to low gastric pH in an attempt to increase gastric acid output. The most common cause of appropriate hypergastrinemia is chronic use of anti-secretory therapy including PPIs and high-dose H2-R antagonists. In approximately one-third of patients on chronic treatment, PPIs have been implicated in elevated FSG levels as high as five times the upper limit of normal [5, 18]. Atrophic gastritis is another common cause of appropriate hypergastrinemia that develops in response to hypo- or achlorhydria [21, 22]. It should be stressed that the level of hypergastrinemia is not discriminatory without identifying the appropriateness of gastric secretion.

ZES is the prototypical cause for inappropriate hypergastrinemia. Gastrin is normally secreted by G-cells in the gastric antrum and regulated by feedback inhibition via paracrine release of somatostatin from adjacent D-cells in the presence of a low gastric pH [23]. Patients with exogenous sources of gastrin (i.e., gastrinomas) are unresponsive to these inhibitory mechanisms, leading to unopposed gastrin release and subsequent gastric acid hypersecretion [24]. In addition to ZES, there are a number of other causes of inappropriate hypergastrinemia that should be considered in any patient prior to intervention. The retained antrum syndrome, in which a cuff of G-cell-containing antrum is retained away from the pathway of gastric acid production, should always be considered in individuals who have undergone prior peptic ulcer surgery (Billroth 2-type resections). Importantly, *H. pylori* infection has been reported to cause both appropriate and inappropriate hypergastrinemia [25] depending on the extent of its mucosal involvement. Antral-predominant infection impairs D-cell somatostatin release, causing a loss of G-cell inhibition and consequently inappropriate hypergastrinemia. The resultant gastric acid hypersecretion can predispose patients to duodenal ulcer disease that can closely mimic ZES [26]. Alternatively, *H. pylori* infection can also cause a pangastritis that leads to gastric acid hyposecretion and consequently appropriate hypergastrinemia [25].

4.3.2 Diagnostic Algorithm for ZES

Once a diagnosis of ZES is suspected, the FSG and assessment of acid secretory capability can be interpreted as is shown in our approach to diagnosis in Fig. 4.2. An elevated FSG is found in >97 % of ZES patients [27]. Although it is rare, gastrin levels have been noted to normalize in ZES patients in two specific scenarios: after gastrinoma resection even in the absence of cure and in MEN-1-associated ZES patients after parathyroidectomy [17, 28]. That being said, in the rare case where strong clinical suspicion for ZES remains despite a normal FSG, diagnosis can be pursued by means of gastrin measurement in response to secretin infusion (Secretin Stimulation Testing [SST]) and BAO measurement. In patients with an elevated FSG, hypergastrinemia secondary to chronic PPI or high-dose H2-R antagonist therapy (i.e., appropriate hypergastrinemia) should be ruled out by a careful wean of anti-secretory medications. It should be stressed that PPI withdrawal in patients with possible ZES is a potentially dangerous intervention that needs to be performed carefully [20, 29–32] and only after complete healing of peptic ulcers. We recommend a slow wean making use of PPIs, H2-R antagonists, and antacids to reduce the risk of severe rebound hypersecretion and possible complications of PUD [19]. During this wean, patients need to maintain strict compliance with the prescribed anti-secretory regimen. It is generally believed that PPIs should be withdrawn for at least a week to restore normal levels of gastric acid production, allowing for accurate measurements of both FSG and gastric pH. Given their shorter duration of action, H2-R antagonists can be used as a replacement for PPIs until 24–30 h prior to testing. During these last 24–30 h, patients may use antacids as needed until midnight the night before their formal testing. Proper anticipatory guidance is necessary and patients should be informed to present to the emergency room should they develop nausea, vomiting, diarrhea, or abdominal pain for prompt nasogastric aspiration. The aspiration of nasogastric contents, as opposed to restarting anti-secretory medications, will render them safe while also preventing a delay in the necessary scheduled testing.

Should the elevated FSG persist after a proper wean of anti-secretory therapy, the concurrently measured gastric pH provides diagnostic categorization (Fig. 4.2). Approximately 99 % of ZES patients have a fasting gastric pH of less than 2 [33]. Thus, in patients with hypergastrinemia and a pH less than 2, ZES is virtually confirmed (in the absence of the retained antrum syndrome) and beginning an assessment of the patient's MEN-1 status and staging with cross-sectional and nuclear imaging is recommended. In those with a concurrently measured gastric pH > 5, ZES is unlikely and an alternative cause for hypergastrinemia should be pursued.

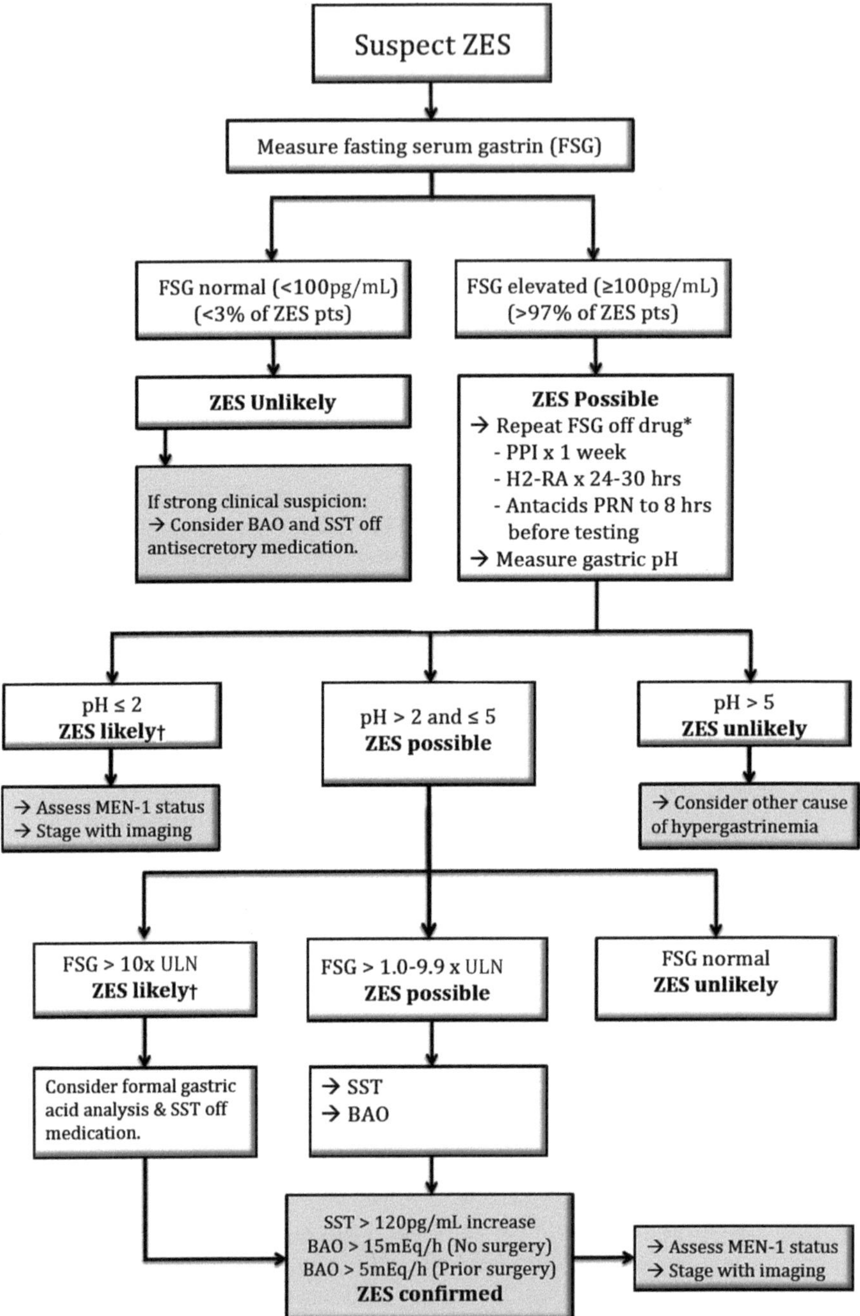

Fig. 4.2 *Algorithm for the diagnosis of Zollinger–Ellison syndrome*. *Weaning patients with possible ZES off antisecretory therapy is a potentially dangerous intervention and should be performed under controlled circumstances preferably in a center with experience. †Exclude retained gastric antrum syndrome. Abbreviations: *ULN*, upper limit of normal, *SST*, secretin stimulation test; *BAO*, basal acid output; *ZES*, Zollinger–Ellison syndrome; *PPI*, Proton pump inhibitor; *H2-RA*, histamine-2 receptor antagonist

In cases where gastric pH falls within the non-diagnostic range (pH>2 and ≤5), ZES remains possible and should be confirmed by SST and BAO measurement. A BAO of greater than 15 mEq/h in the presence of any level of hypergastrinemia is pathognomonic of ZES. A secretin stimulation test with an increase of greater than 120 pg/mL was recently shown to have the greatest sensitivity (94 %) and specificity (100 %) for ZES [34]; however, increases of greater than 110–220 pg/mL have also been used previously [29, 35, 36]. In the past, the calcium infusion test was performed as a confirmatory test, but this has been abandoned due to the potential for complications. Until recently, gastric acid analysis for the diagnosis of ZES was further honed by measuring the maximal secretory capacity of the stomach (maximal acid output [MAO]) after stimulation with subcutaneous pentagastrin (or, before this, with histamine agonists) [33, 37]; however, pharmacologic gastric stimulants are no longer available in the United States despite their potential role to improve diagnostic yield [38].

It is important to note several studies have questioned the accuracy of diagnostic testing for ZES. In a recent study, a majority of commercial kits tested were found to inaccurately measure plasma concentrations of gastrin due to the use of antibodies with inappropriate specificity [39]. In regards to SST, it is now well accepted that chronic PPI treatment or hypo- or achlorhydria can result in false positive results [40–44]. Thus, it is important to interpret results of this test in the context of a patient's gastric acid secretory status.

4.3.3 Tumor Markers

Gastrin, the tumor marker of choice for diagnosis, is present in many forms in the serum of ZES patients. Gastrinomas primarily release fully processed amidated gastrins (gastrin-17 and gastrin-34), but may also secrete a range of gastrin precursors including prograstrin and various COOH glycine-extended forms [5, 45–48]. The ability of a gastrinoma to produce and secrete any of a range of potential gastrin peptides explains the inaccuracy of some commercial gastrin kits as was discussed above—several with high rates of false negatives were found to use antibodies binding exclusively to gastrin-17 (see Table 4.3, "Spurious Hypergastrinemia").

In addition to gastrin, gastrinomas, like other gastrointestinal and pancreatic neuroendocrine tumors, frequently secrete multiple peptides that can function as tumor markers including chromogranin A and B, neuron-specific enolase, and pancreatic polypeptide [5, 49, 50]. These markers do not play a significant role in diagnosis but serial marker measurements (particularly chromogranin A) may be useful for monitoring gastrinoma growth and disease extent according to some [51–55] but not other investigators [50].

A novel biomarker derived from chromogranins, pancreastatin, has recently been shown to rise in the setting of neuroendocrine tumors independent of PPI use and may become an option in these patients that would preclude the need for PPI cessation; however, its use in the setting of gastrinoma diagnosis requires further testing [56, 57].

4.3.4 Tumor Localization Strategies

Once the diagnosis of ZES has been established, tumor localization is necessary to assist in determining tumor location, disease extent, and presence of liver involvement to plan treatment. A number of localization methods have been recommended including conventional cross-sectional imaging studies (computed tomography [CT], magnetic resonance imaging [MRI], ultrasonography), nuclear imaging (somatostatin receptor scintigraphy [SRS]), functional localization strategies (selective arteriography and intra-arterial secretin stimulation with venous measurement of gastrin gradients), as well as endoscopic ultrasound. The results of a prospective study of 80 patients with ZES to determine the sensitivity of these tumor localization studies are shown in Table 4.4 [58]. Due to the high density of surface somatostatin receptors present on gastrinomas [59], SRS is one of the most sensitive tests for the localization of both primary and metastatic gastrinomas with a sensitivity of ~70 %; a number that rivals that of using all conventional imaging studies combined (59 %) and which is significantly higher than each one individually (range 19–45 %) [58]. Thus, SRS is currently recommended as the imaging modality of choice for both localizing a primary tumor as well as determining disease extent at diagnosis and during follow-up. The use of novel PET tracers such as ^{68}Gallium-tagged somatostatin analogs (^{68}Gallium DOTANOC, DOTATOC, and DOTATATE) in somatostatin receptor positron emission tomography (PET) and PET/CT has been shown to improve on the sensitivity of standard SRS in a recent meta-analysis (Table 4.4, Fig. 4.3) [60]; however, its use is currently limited to specialized centers.

To further assist in treatment decisions, cross-sectional anatomic imaging with a triple-phase CT or an MRI scan with gadolinium enhancement is also recommended to supplement SRS with information regarding exact tumor location and size (modern SRS includes fusion imaging with CT scanning to provide some additional anatomical information but at low resolution only). Endoscopic ultrasound (discussed

Table 4.4 Sensitivity of tumor localization modalities in patients with ZES

Tumor localization modality	Sensitivity (%)	*p* value
Ultrasonography (US)	19	<0.001
Computed tomography (CT)	38	<0.001
Magnetic resonance imaging (MRI)	45	<0.001
Angiography	40	<0.001
Any of US, CT, MRI, or Angiography	59	>0.05
Somatostatin Receptor Scintigraphy (SRS)	70	–
SRS + All other tests	75	–
^{68}Gallium SRS[a]	93	–

p value for the method compared to SRS alone. $N=80$ consecutive patients with ZES. Data from Gibril et al. (1996)

[a]Data from Treglia et al. (2012). Pooled data from $N=567$ patients

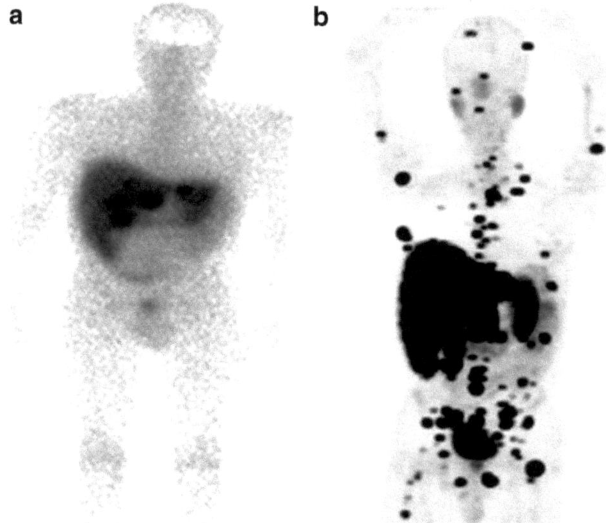

Fig. 4.3 *Comparison of somatostatin receptor-based imaging modalities.* A comparison of (**a**) ^{111}Indium SRS in the evaluation of a patient with metastatic gastrinoma and (**b**) ^{68}Galium SRS in the same patient within 2 months. ^{68}Galium SRS has been shown to improve on the sensitivity of standard SRS and procures higher resolution images due to greater receptor affinity of ^{68}Galium tagged tracers

in detail in Chaps. 8 and 14) is useful for localizing primary pancreatic tumors, but frequently misses both duodenal gastrinomas and liver metastases [61–63].

4.4 Management of ZES

4.4.1 Control of Gastric Acid Hypersecretion

Prior to the development of histamine H2-R antagonists and then PPIs, patients with ZES were at major risk of succumbing to the complications of uncontrolled PUD. For these patients, the mainstay of treatment was total gastrectomy. The development of PPIs has allowed for effective control of gastric acid hypersecretion in almost every patient [64, 65] such that the use of this aggressive and potentially morbid surgery is now reserved only for the rare patient (<0.5 %) who cannot tolerate or is refractory to PPI therapy [66–68].

When initiating PPIs, higher doses than those that are usually prescribed for idiopathic acid-peptic disorders given twice daily for both sporadic and MEN-1-associated disease are generally recommended—40 mg twice daily for omeprazole, esomeprazole, rabeprazole, and pantoprazole or 30 mg twice daily for lansoprazole.

Lower doses (20 mg/day) have been shown to fall short of controlling the symptoms of ZES patients [69] and therefore, are not expected to allow for proper healing of peptic ulcers. For patients with MEN-1-associated ZES, surgical correction of hyperparathyroidism should be targeted as this has been associated with a decline in both FSG level and BAO as well as increased sensitivity to anti-secretory drugs [17, 28]. The goal of treatment is to reduce acid hypersecretion as measured by BAO<10 mEq/h in the last hour before the next dose of drug in patients without previous gastric acid-reducing surgery and <5 mEq/h in patients with prior surgery to allow for healing of PUD and to prevent recurrence [65, 68, 70].

ZES patients have been treated with PPIs for greater than 20 years without significant side effects or evidence of tachyphylaxis; on the contrary, most patients can safely reduce their dosing over time while maintaining effective control of symptoms and acid secretory capability [65]. However, we generally advocate long-term twice daily dosing schedules in patients with persistent disease to prevent a sudden loss of control of acid output with potentially life-threatening consequences in the event that a dose is inadvertently missed or malabsorbed. A reduction in vitamin B_{12} levels has been reported with long-term PPI use; however, it does not appear to affect body iron stores as previously theorized [67, 71, 72].

4.4.2 Surgical Management of Gastrinoma

With the control of gastric acid production provided by PPIs, the natural history of the tumor itself is now the main determinant of long-term survival. As was previously mentioned, 60–90 % of gastrinomas are believed to be malignant [5] with one large study identifying that up to 25 % show especially rapid growth associated with poor 10-year survival [7].

With a greater proportion of patients now dying from the malignant nature of their gastrinoma [7, 73], studies over the last two decades have focused on surgical means of delaying metastases and offering cure. Surgery has been shown to decrease the development of liver metastasis [61, 74], potentially improve survival, and produce long-term cure in up to 40 % of patients [29, 61, 75–78]. In addition, gastrinomas almost always develop within an anatomic boundary known as the triangle of Stabile [6], represented in Fig. 4.4 with a majority found within the duodenum (Fig. 4.5a). This predictability allows surgeons to perform exploratory surgery for resection in patients even with negative imaging studies. Thus, routine surgical exploration with curative intent is recommended in cases of localized disease in sporadic patients who lack other medical comorbidities that increase surgical risk or shorten life expectancy.

At surgery, enucleation of the pancreatic head or body lesions is recommended and if necessary, distal pancreatectomy for pancreatic tail lesions near the spleen. Duodenotomy is a standard component of gastrinoma surgery because it is essential to localize small duodenal tumors that may be missed on cross-sectional imaging [76, 78, 79]. In addition, intraoperative ultrasound and endoscopic transillumination

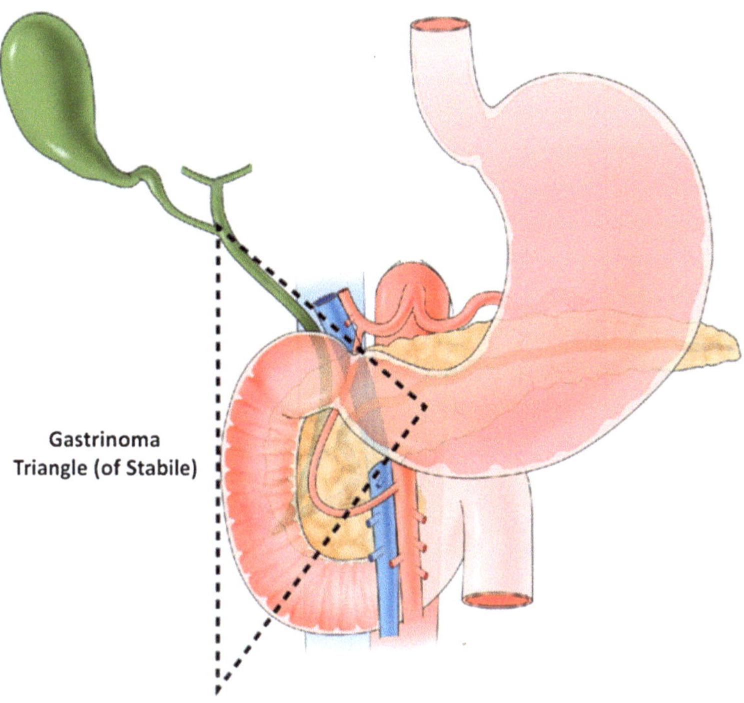

Fig. 4.4 *Gastrinoma Triangle*. Most gastrinomas are found within the Gastrinoma Triangle (of Stabile), an anatomic boundary formed by the junction of the common and cystic ducts (superiorly), the junction of the second and third segments of the duodenum (inferiorly), and the intersection of the head and neck of the pancreas (medially). Most sporadic gastrinomas arise in the duodenal wall. *Reproduced with permission from Elsevier Limited, Metz (2012)*

of the duodenum at surgery is also recommended to assist in localization of duodenal tumors and optimal placement of the duodenotomy [79]. Furthermore, regional lymph node dissection is mandatory necessitating open (as opposed to laparoscopic) surgery for a ZES exploration. Recent data indicates that the likelihood of a biochemical cure is higher in patients without nodal disease than in those with lymph node involvement [80]. After apparently curative resection (i.e., resolution of inappropriate hypergastrinemia and negative imaging studies), patients should be evaluated with both periodic FSG measurements as well as SST with cross-sectional imaging being reserved for cases of biochemical recurrence. During this time, acid-secretory therapy should be maintained and only weaned if there is evidence of a biochemical cure without symptoms. After curative resection, reversal of gastric acid hypersecretion takes up to 6 months and does not normalize in all patients [81].

The role for surgery in MEN-1 patients is controversial as these patients develop multiple tumors [3] (Fig. 4.5) and are rarely, if ever, cured of ZES without radical surgery, which is associated with post-operative morbidity in approximately 40 % of patients [82, 83]. Surgical management of these patients is directed at delaying liver

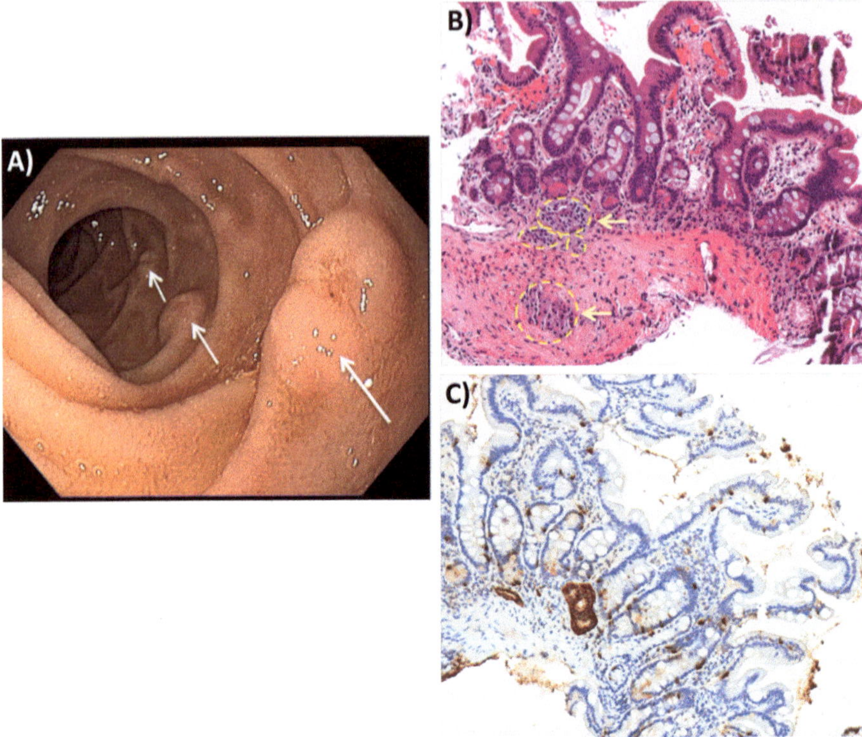

Fig. 4.5 *Multiple duodenal gastrinomas in a patient with MEN-1-associated ZES.* (**a**) In MEN-1-associated ZES, patients commonly develop multiple tumors within the duodenum (*white arrows*) and pancreas. (**b**) Histologic sections show a focus of well-differentiated neuroendocrine tumor (*yellow arrows*) involving duodenal mucosa and muscularis mucosa (hematoxylin-eosin, original magnification × 150). Note the tumor lies below the epithelial layer; therefore, the overlying mucosa may appear normal on endoscopy. (**c**) A chromogranin stain highlights the neuroendocrine tumor (chromogranin, original magnification × 150). *Images attributed to Melissa Grilliot, MD, Department of Pathology, Hospital of the University of Pennsylvania*

metastasis, a poor prognostic indicator [7, 73, 80, 84–87]. In the MEN-1 population, the current surgical recommendations vary and include resection of pancreatic masses with sizes greater than 2.0–2.5 cm [79] and 3.0 cm [88, 89], citing studies linking tumor size to risk of liver metastasis. Other groups avoid surgery altogether choosing instead to control gastric acid hypersecretion alone [31, 90, 91]. Most, but not all [31, 92, 93], of the current surgical recommendations reflect extensive research from the NIH [4, 7, 33, 73, 75–77] and therefore may not be directly applicable to tertiary care centers managing these patients according to different protocols.

By extrapolating from data derived from patients with metastatic carcinoid tumors [94], surgery may also have a role in metastatic sporadic disease where the aim is to debulk tumor and potentially improve outcome by slowing the progression of liver disease and development of more distant metastases. This approach may be

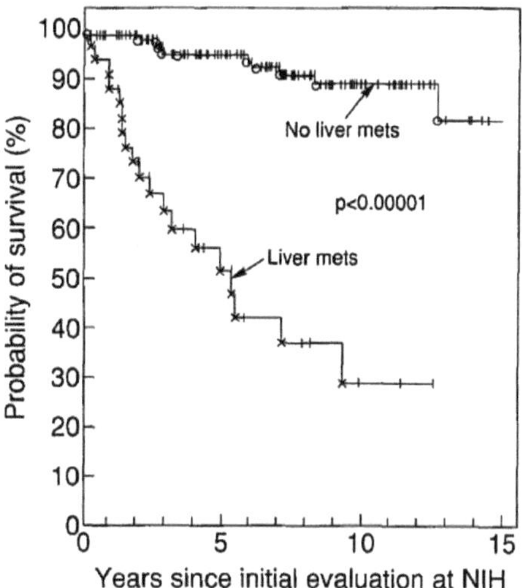

Fig. 4.6 *Comparison of survival curves based on presence of liver metastases.* Comparison of the survival curves between ZES patients with or without liver metastases calculated from initial admission data plotted in the form of Kaplan-Meier, $N = 185$. *Reproduced with permission from Elsevier Limited, Weber et al. (1995)*

of specific value in patients whose primary tumors are in situ as both locations can potentially be addressed simultaneously. In contrast, if the primary is already out, liver-directed therapy with interventional radiological techniques (see below) is potentially more practical. Finally, liver transplantation is an option in only a small, select group of patients and it is not generally considered standard therapy for metastatic neuroendocrine tumors.

4.4.3 Medical Management of Advanced Disease

In the majority of patients who are not cured by surgical resection or not deemed surgical candidates due to unresectable disease or comorbidities, there is a developing armamentarium of multi-disciplinary therapies that can be offered. These treatments target those with liver metastases, a particularly poor prognostic feature (Fig. 4.6). Ten-year survival in ZES patients without liver involvement approaches 96 %, but declines rapidly with the development of limited metastases (78–80 %) and further still for patients with diffuse liver involvement (16 %) [73].

For these patients, long-acting somatostatin analogs such as ocreotide acetate LAR and lanreotide SR are recommended first-line antitumor treatments. In general, therapy with these agents is only considered after the demonstration of increasing tumor bulk on imaging. These agents have been shown to reduce tumor-related symptoms and produce an enduring antitumor effect with tumoristasis in 40–70 % [95, 96] and tumor regression in ~10 % of patients. In the PROMID study of 85 patients with well-differentiated metastatic midgut neuroendocrine tumors, octreotide LAR (30 mg subcutaneously per month) was shown to improve median progression free survival (14.3 months vs. 6 months), but did not note any difference in median overall survival [97]. Given their focused therapeutic target, these treatments have a relatively benign side effect profile that includes nausea, abdominal pain, diarrhea, gallstone formation, and glucose intolerance. These reported side effects are generally acceptable for patients and short-lived in most cases [95, 98].

For patients with growing or symptomatic liver metastases, a patent portal vein, and no evidence of distant disease, selective embolization or chemoembolization via the hepatic artery is the preferred method of regional treatment. This treatment, which can be repeated at intervals providing that vascular access is maintained, can improve tumor-related symptoms, but has not been shown to prolong survival. An alternative method of administering liver-directed therapy is with radioactive Yttrium beads (Sir-Spheres microspheres, Sirtex, Woburn, MA, USA or TheraSphere, Nordion, Ottawa, Ontario, Canada). This therapy has not been compared with embolization techniques directly but the two methods are likely of similar efficacy and may well be complementary.

Recently, the FDA approved two new small molecule targeted therapies for the management of patients with metastatic pancreatic neuroendocrine tumors, everolimus [99, 100], an mTOR inhibitor, and sunitinib [101], a VEGF inhibitor. While studies in gastrinoma, specifically, have yet to be done, it is likely that these agents will play a role in the management of widely metastatic ZES. In comparison, older chemotherapy regimens with streptozocin and doxorubicin with or without 5-fluorouracil have been shown to decrease tumor size in up to 50 % of patients but they have not been shown to extend survival and are associated with considerable organ toxicity [27]. These agents should only be considered in patients with rapidly growing diffuse liver metastases that fail other directed treatments. More recently, Strosberg et al. [101] published a retrospective study of 30 patients with metastatic pancreatic neuroendocrine tumors treated with a combination of capecitabine and temozolomide (CAPTEM). This treatment was associated with superior response rates, survival, and toxicity when compared to streptozocin-based regimens [102] and is currently being investigated in a phase II clinical trial.

Finally, the overexpression of somatostatin receptors on gastrinomas has become the molecular basis for the use of ^{90}Yttrium and ^{177}Lutetium-based peptide receptor radionuclide therapy (PRRT). Preliminary studies have shown PRRT to be an effective antitumor therapy [103]; however, larger, long-term studies of its use in the context of other treatment options are necessary to better define its use.

References

1. Zollinger RM, Ellison EH. Primary peptic ulcerations of the jejunum associated with islet cell tumors of the pancreas. Ann Surg. 1955;142(4):709–23. discussion, 24-8. Epub 1955/10/01.
2. Gibril F, Jensen RT. Zollinger-Ellison syndrome revisited: diagnosis, biologic markers, associated inherited disorders, and acid hypersecretion. Curr Gastroenterol Rep. 2004;6(6):454–63. Epub 2004/11/06.
3. Pipeleers-Marichal M, Somers G, Willems G, Foulis A, Imrie C, Bishop AE, et al. Gastrinomas in the duodenums of patients with multiple endocrine neoplasia type 1 and the Zollinger-Ellison syndrome. N Engl J Med. 1990;322(11):723–7. Epub 1990/03/15.

4. Roy PK, Venzon DJ, Shojamanesh H, Abou-Saif A, Peghini P, Doppman JL, et al. Zollinger-Ellison syndrome. Clinical presentation in 261 patients. Medicine (Baltimore). 2000;79(6):379–411. Epub 2001/01/06.
5. Jensen RT, Norton JA. Pancreatic endocrine neoplasms. In: Fordtran JS, Sleisenger MH, Feldman M, Scharschmidt BF, editors. Gastrointestinal diseases: pathophysiology, diagnosis and management. 2nd ed. Philadelphia: Saunders; 1993.
6. Stabile BE, Morrow DJ, Passaro Jr E. The gastrinoma triangle: operative implications. Am J Surg. 1984;147(1):25–31. Epub 1984/01/01.
7. Weber HC, Venzon DJ, Lin JT, Fishbein VA, Orbuch M, Strader DB, et al. Determinants of metastatic rate and survival in patients with Zollinger-Ellison syndrome: a prospective long-term study. Gastroenterology. 1995;108(6):1637–49. Epub 1995/06/01.
8. Waxman I, Gardner JD, Jensen RT, Maton PN. Peptic ulcer perforation as the presentation of Zollinger-Ellison syndrome. Dig Dis Sci. 1991;36(1):19–24. Epub 1991/01/01.
9. Locke 3rd GR, Talley NJ, Fett SL, Zinsmeister AR, Melton 3rd LJ. Prevalence and clinical spectrum of gastroesophageal reflux: a population-based study in Olmsted County, Minnesota. Gastroenterology. 1997;112(5):1448–56. Epub 1997/05/01.
10. Benya RV, Metz DC, Venzon DJ, Fishbeyn VA, Strader DB, Orbuch M, et al. Zollinger-Ellison syndrome can be the initial endocrine manifestation in patients with multiple endocrine neoplasia-type I. Am J Med. 1994;97(5):436–44. Epub 1994/11/01.
11. Thompson JC, Reeder DD, Villar HV, Fender HR. Natural history and experience with diagnosis and treatment of the Zollinger-Ellison syndrome. Surg Gynecol Obstet. 1975;140(5):721–39. Epub 1975/05/01.
12. Kaplan EL, Horvath K, Udekwu A, Straus 2nd F, Schark C, Ferguson DJ, et al. Gastrinomas: a 42-year experience. World J Surg. 1990;14(3):365–75. discussion 75-6. Epub 1990/05/01.
13. Soga J, Yakuwa Y. The gastrinoma/Zollinger-Ellison syndrome: statistical evaluation of a Japanese series of 359 cases. J Hepatobiliary Pancreat Surg. 1998;5(1):77–85. Epub 1998/07/31.
14. Farley DR, van Heerden JA, Grant CS, Miller LJ, Ilstrup DM. The Zollinger-Ellison syndrome. A collective surgical experience. Ann Surg. 1992;215(6):561–9. discussion 9-70. Epub 1992/06/01.
15. Miller LS, Vinayek R, Frucht H, Gardner JD, Jensen RT, Maton PN. Reflux esophagitis in patients with Zollinger-Ellison syndrome. Gastroenterology. 1990;98(2):341–6. Epub 1990/02/01.
16. Weber HC, Venzon DJ, Jensen RT, Metz DC. Studies on the interrelation between Zollinger-Ellison syndrome, Helicobacter pylori, and proton pump inhibitor therapy. Gastroenterology. 1997;112(1):84–91. Epub 1997/01/01.
17. Jensen RT. Management of the Zollinger-Ellison syndrome in patients with multiple endocrine neoplasia type 1. J Intern Med. 1998;243(6):477–88. Epub 1998/07/29.
18. Corleto VD, Annibale B, Gibril F, Angeletti S, Serrano J, Venzon DJ, et al. Does the widespread use of proton pump inhibitors mask, complicate and/or delay the diagnosis of Zollinger-Ellison syndrome? Aliment Pharmacol Ther. 2001;15(10):1555–61. Epub 2001/09/21.
19. Metz DC. Diagnosis of the Zollinger-Ellison syndrome. Clin Gastroenterol Hepatol. 2012;10(2):126–30. Epub 2011/08/03.
20. Metz DC, Jensen RT. Gastrointestinal neuroendocrine tumors: pancreatic endocrine tumors. Gastroenterology. 2008;135(5):1469–92. Epub 2008/08/16.
21. Annibale B, Marignani M, Azzoni C, D'Ambra G, Caruana P, D'Adda T, et al. Atrophic body gastritis: distinct features associated with Helicobacter pylori infection. Helicobacter. 1997;2(2):57–64. Epub 1997/06/01.
22. Asaka M, Kato M, Kudo M, Katagiri M, Nishikawa K, Koshiyama H, et al. Atrophic changes of gastric mucosa are caused by Helicobacter pylori infection rather than aging: studies in asymptomatic Japanese adults. Helicobacter. 1996;1(1):52–6. Epub 1996/03/01.
23. Wolfe MM, Reel GM, McGuigan JE. Inhibition of gastrin release by secretin is mediated by somatostatin in cultured rat antral mucosa. J Clin Invest. 1983;72(5):1586–93. Epub 1983/11/01.

24. Maton P, Dayal Y. Clinical implications of hypergastrinemia. In: Zakim D, Dannenberg A, editors. Peptic ulcer disease and other acid-related disorders. Armonk, NY: Academic Research; 1991. p. 213.
25. McColl KE, el-Omar E, Gillen D. Interactions between H. pylori infection, gastric acid secretion and anti-secretory therapy. Br Med Bull. 1998;54(1):121–38.
26. Metz DC, Weber HC, Orbuch M, Strader DB, Lubensky IA, Jensen RT. Helicobacter pylori infection. A reversible cause of hypergastrinemia and hyperchlorhydria which may mimic Zollinger-Ellison syndrome. Dig Dis Sci. 1995;40(1):153–9. Epub 1995/01/01.
27. Jensen RT. Gastrinomas: advances in diagnosis and management. Neuroendocrinology. 2004;80 Suppl 1:23–7. Epub 2004/10/13.
28. Norton JA, Cornelius MJ, Doppman JL, Maton PN, Gardner JD, Jensen RT. Effect of parathyroidectomy in patients with hyperparathyroidism, Zollinger-Ellison syndrome, and multiple endocrine neoplasia type I: a prospective study. Surgery. 1987;102(6):958–66. Epub 1987/12/01.
29. Fishbeyn VA, Norton JA, Benya RV, Pisegna JR, Venzon DJ, Metz DC, et al. Assessment and prediction of long-term cure in patients with the Zollinger-Ellison syndrome: the best approach. Ann Intern Med. 1993;119(3):199–206. Epub 1993/08/01.
30. Poitras P, Gingras MH, Rehfeld JF. The Zollinger-Ellison syndrome: dangers and consequences of interrupting antisecretory treatment. Clin Gastroenterol Hepatol. 2012;10(2): 199–202. Epub 2011/08/30.
31. Wilcox CM, Seay T, Arcury JT, Mohnen J, Hirschowitz BI. Zollinger-Ellison syndrome: presentation, response to therapy, and outcome. Dig Liver Dis. 2011;43(6):439–43. Epub 2011/01/05.
32. Dhillo WS, Jayasena CN, Lewis CJ, Martin NM, Tang KC, Meeran K, et al. Plasma gastrin measurement cannot be used to diagnose a gastrinoma in patients on either proton pump inhibitors or histamine type-2 receptor antagonists. Ann Clin Biochem. 2006;43(Pt 2):153–5. Epub 2006/03/16.
33. Roy PK, Venzon DJ, Feigenbaum KM, Koviack PD, Bashir S, Ojeaburu JV, et al. Gastric secretion in Zollinger-Ellison syndrome. Correlation with clinical expression, tumor extent and role in diagnosis—a prospective NIH study of 235 patients and a review of 984 cases in the literature. Medicine (Baltimore). 2001;80(3):189–222. Epub 2001/06/05.
34. Berna MJ, Hoffmann KM, Long SH, Serrano J, Gibril F, Jensen RT. Serum gastrin in Zollinger-Ellison syndrome: II. Prospective study of gastrin provocative testing in 293 patients from the National Institutes of Health and comparison with 537 cases from the literature. Evaluation of diagnostic criteria, proposal of new criteria, and correlations with clinical and tumoral features. Medicine (Baltimore). 2006;85(6):331–64. Epub 2006/11/17.
35. Metz DC, Buchanan M, Purich E, Fein S. A randomized controlled crossover study comparing synthetic porcine and human secretins with biologically derived porcine secretin to diagnose Zollinger-Ellison syndrome. Aliment Pharmacol Ther. 2001;15(5):669–76. Epub 2001/05/01.
36. Frucht H, Howard JM, Slaff JI, Wank SA, McCarthy DM, Maton PN, et al. Secretin and calcium provocative tests in the Zollinger-Ellison syndrome. A prospective study. Ann Intern Med. 1989;111(9):713–22. Epub 1989/11/01.
37. Wolfe MM, Jensen RT. Zollinger-Ellison syndrome. Current concepts in diagnosis and management. N Engl J Med. 1987;317(19):1200–9. Epub 1987/11/05.
38. Metz DC, Starr JA. A retrospective study of the usefulness of acid secretory testing. Aliment Pharmacol Ther. 2000;14(1):103–11. Epub 2000/01/13.
39. Rehfeld JF, Gingras MH, Bardram L, Hilsted L, Goetze JP, Poitras P. The Zollinger-Ellison syndrome and mismeasurement of gastrin. Gastroenterology. 2011;140(5):1444–53. Epub 2011/02/15.
40. Brady 3rd CE, Utts SJ, Dev J. False-positive gastrin rises after secretin injection. J Lab Clin Med. 1985;106(4):461–2. Epub 1985/10/01.
41. Feldman M, Schiller LR, Walsh JH, Fordtran JS, Richardson CT. Positive intravenous secretin test in patients with achlorhydria-related hypergastrinemia. Gastroenterology. 1987; 93(1):59–62. Epub 1987/07/01.

42. Goldman JA, Blanton WP, Hay DW, Wolfe MM. False-positive secretin stimulation test for gastrinoma associated with the use of proton pump inhibitor therapy. Clin Gastroenterol Hepatol. 2009;7(5):600–2. Epub 2009/02/28.
43. Wollmuth RL, Wagonfeld JB. False-positive secretin test. Ann Intern Med. 1978;88(5):718–9. Epub 1978/05/01.
44. Shah P(1), Singh MH, Yang YX, Metz DC. Hypochlorhydria and achlorhydria are associated with false-positive secretin stimulation testing for Zollinger-Ellison syndrome. Pancreas. 2013;42(6):932–6. doi:10.1097/MPA.0b013e3182847b2e.
45. Rehfeld J, Bardram L. Recent advances in research and management. Endocrine tumors of the pancreas. Basel: S. Karger; 1995. p. 84–98.
46. Rehfeld JF, van Solinge WW. The tumor biology of gastrin and cholecystokinin. Adv Cancer Res. 1994;63:295–347. Epub 1994/01/01.
47. Bardram L. Progastrin in pancreas and the Zollinger-Ellison syndrome. Scand J Gastroenterol. 1990;25(12):1185–95. Epub 1990/12/01.
48. Bardram L. Progastrin in serum from Zollinger-Ellison patients. An indicator of malignancy? Gastroenterology. 1990;98(6):1420–6.
49. Chiang HC, O'Dorisio TM, Huang SC, Maton PN, Gardner JD, Jensen RT. Multiple hormone elevations in Zollinger-Ellison syndrome. Prospective study of clinical significance and of the development of a second symptomatic pancreatic endocrine tumor syndrome. Gastroenterology. 1990;99(6):1565–75. Epub 1990/12/01.
50. Abou-Saif A, Gibril F, Ojeaburu JV, Bashir S, Entsuah LK, Asgharian B, et al. Prospective study of the ability of serial measurements of serum chromogranin A and gastrin to detect changes in tumor burden in patients with gastrinomas. Cancer. 2003;98(2):249–61. Epub 2003/07/23.
51. Bajetta E, Ferrari L, Martinetti A, Celio L, Procopio G, Artale S, et al. Chromogranin A, neuron specific enolase, carcinoembryonic antigen, and hydroxyindole acetic acid evaluation in patients with neuroendocrine tumors. Cancer. 1999;86(5):858–65. Epub 1999/08/27.
52. Goebel SU, Serrano J, Yu F, Gibril F, Venzon DJ, Jensen RT. Prospective study of the value of serum chromogranin A or serum gastrin levels in the assessment of the presence, extent, or growth of gastrinomas. Cancer. 1999;85(7):1470–83. Epub 1999/04/08.
53. Nobels FR, Kwekkeboom DJ, Coopmans W, Schoenmakers CH, Lindemans J, De Herder WW, et al. Chromogranin A as serum marker for neuroendocrine neoplasia: comparison with neuron-specific enolase and the alpha-subunit of glycoprotein hormones. J Clin Endocrinol Metab. 1997;82(8):2622–8. Epub 1997/08/01.
54. Peracchi M, Conte D, Gebbia C, Penati C, Pizzinelli S, Arosio M, et al. Plasma chromogranin A in patients with sporadic gastro-entero-pancreatic neuroendocrine tumors or multiple endocrine neoplasia type 1. Eur J Endocrinol. 2003;148(1):39–43. Epub 2003/01/22.
55. Taupenot L, Harper KL, O'Connor DT. The chromogranin-secretogranin family. N Engl J Med. 2003;348(12):1134–49. Epub 2003/03/21.
56. Ito T, Igarashi H, Jensen RT. Serum pancreastatin: the long sought universal, sensitive, specific tumor marker for neuroendocrine tumors? Pancreas. 2012;41(4):505–7. Epub 2012/04/17.
57. Raines D, Chester M, Diebold AE, Mamikunian P, Anthony CT, Mamikunian G, et al. A prospective evaluation of the effect of chronic proton pump inhibitor use on plasma biomarker levels in humans. Pancreas. 2012;41(4):508–11. Epub 2012/03/31.
58. Gibril F, Reynolds JC, Doppman JL, Chen CC, Venzon DJ, Termanini B, et al. Somatostatin receptor scintigraphy: its sensitivity compared with that of other imaging methods in detecting primary and metastatic gastrinomas. A prospective study. Ann Intern Med. 1996;125(1):26–34. Epub 1996/07/01.
59. Reubi JC, Hacki WH, Lamberts SW. Hormone-producing gastrointestinal tumors contain a high density of somatostatin receptors. J Clin Endocrinol Metab. 1987;65(6):1127–34. Epub 1987/12/01.
60. Treglia G, Castaldi P, Rindi G, Giordano A, Rufini V. Diagnostic performance of Gallium-68 somatostatin receptor PET and PET/CT in patients with thoracic and gastroenteropancreatic neuroendocrine tumours: a meta-analysis. Endocrine. 2012;42(1):80–7. Epub 2012/02/22.

61. Norton JA, Alexander HR, Fraker DL, Venzon DJ, Gibril F, Jensen RT. Does the use of routine duodenotomy (DUODX) affect rate of cure, development of liver metastases, or survival in patients with Zollinger-Ellison syndrome? Ann Surg. 2004;239(5):617–25. discussion 26. Epub 2004/04/15.
62. Ruszniewski P, Amouyal P, Amouyal G, Grange JD, Mignon M, Bouche O, et al. Localization of gastrinomas by endoscopic ultrasonography in patients with Zollinger-Ellison syndrome. Surgery. 1995;117(6):629–35. Epub 1995/06/01.
63. Anderson MA, Carpenter S, Thompson NW, Nostrant TT, Elta GH, Scheiman JM. Endoscopic ultrasound is highly accurate and directs management in patients with neuroendocrine tumors of the pancreas. Am J Gastroenterol. 2000;95(9):2271–7. Epub 2000/09/28.
64. Maton PN, Vinayek R, Frucht H, McArthur KA, Miller LS, Saeed ZA, et al. Long-term efficacy and safety of omeprazole in patients with Zollinger-Ellison syndrome: a prospective study. Gastroenterology. 1989;97(4):827–36. Epub 1989/10/01.
65. Metz DC, Pisegna JR, Fishbeyn VA, Benya RV, Feigenbaum KM, Koviack PD, et al. Currently used doses of omeprazole in Zollinger-Ellison syndrome are too high. Gastroenterology. 1992;103(5):1498–508. Epub 1992/11/01.
66. Wilcox CM, Seay T, Arcury J, Hirschowitz BI. Presentation, response to lansoprazole therapy, and outcome of Zollinger-Ellison syndrome-like gastric acid hypersecretors. Scand J Gastroenterol. 2011;46(3):277–80. Epub 2010/11/16.
67. Hirschowitz BI, Simmons J, Mohnen J. Long-term lansoprazole control of gastric acid and pepsin secretion in ZE and non-ZE hypersecretors: a prospective 10-year study. Aliment Pharmacol Ther. 2001;15(11):1795–806. Epub 2001/10/31.
68. Metz D, Jensen R. Advances in gastric antisecretory therapy in Zollinger-Ellison syndrome. In: Mignon M, Jensen R, editors. Endocrine tumors of the pancreas: recent advances in research and management. Basel: S. Karger; 1995. p. 240–57.
69. Termanini B, Gibril F, Stewart CA, Weber HC, Jensen RT. A prospective study of the effectiveness of low dose omeprazole as initial therapy in Zollinger-Ellison syndrome. Aliment Pharmacol Ther. 1996;10(1):61–71. Epub 1996/02/01.
70. Jensen R, Norton J. Endocrine tumors of the pancreas. In: Yamada T, Alpers BH, Owyang C, Powell DW, Silverstein FE, editors. Textbook of gastroenterology. 2nd ed. Philadelphia: J.B. Lippincot; 1995. p. 2131–66.
71. Metz DC, Pisegna JR, Ringham GL, Feigenbaum K, Koviack PD, Maton PN, et al. Prospective study of efficacy and safety of lansoprazole in Zollinger-Ellison syndrome. Dig Dis Sci. 1993;38(2):245–56. Epub 1993/02/01.
72. Termanini B, Gibril F, Sutliff VE, Yu F, Venzon DJ, Jensen RT. Effect of long-term gastric acid suppressive therapy on serum vitamin B12 levels in patients with Zollinger-Ellison syndrome. Am J Med. 1998;104(5):422–30. Epub 1998/06/17.
73. Yu F, Venzon DJ, Serrano J, Goebel SU, Doppman JL, Gibril F, et al. Prospective study of the clinical course, prognostic factors, causes of death, and survival in patients with long-standing Zollinger-Ellison syndrome. J Clin Oncol. 1999;17(2):615–30. Epub 1999/03/18.
74. Fraker DL, Norton JA, Alexander HR, Venzon DJ, Jensen RT. Surgery in Zollinger-Ellison syndrome alters the natural history of gastrinoma. Ann Surg. 1994;220(3):320–8. discussion 8-30. Epub 1994/09/01.
75. Norton JA, Doppman JL, Jensen RT. Curative resection in Zollinger-Ellison syndrome. Results of a 10-year prospective study. Ann Surg. 1992;215(1):8–18.
76. Norton JA, Fraker DL, Alexander HR, Venzon DJ, Doppman JL, Serrano J, et al. Surgery to cure the Zollinger-Ellison syndrome. N Engl J Med. 1999;341(9):635–44. Epub 1999/08/26.
77. Norton JA, Fraker DL, Alexander HR, Gibril F, Liewehr DJ, Venzon DJ, et al. Surgery increases survival in patients with gastrinoma. Ann Surg. 2006;244(3):410–9. Epub 2006/08/24.
78. Norton JA, Jensen RT. Current surgical management of Zollinger-Ellison syndrome (ZES) in patients without multiple endocrine neoplasia-type 1 (MEN1). Surg Oncol. 2003;12(2):145–51. Epub 2003/08/30.

79. Norton JA, Fang TD, Jensen RT. Surgery for gastrinoma and insulinoma in multiple endocrine neoplasia type 1. J Natl Compr Canc Netw. 2006;4(2):148–53. Epub 2006/02/03.
80. Singh MH, Fraker DL, Metz DC. Importance of surveillance for multiple endocrine neoplasia-1 and surgery in patients with sporadic Zollinger-Ellison syndrome. Clin Gastroenterol Hepatol. 2012;10(11):1262–9. Epub 2012/08/21.
81. Metz DC, Benya RV, Fishbeyn VA, Pisegna JR, Orbuch M, Strader DB, et al. Prospective study of the need for long-term antisecretory therapy in patients with Zollinger-Ellison syndrome following successful curative gastrinoma resection. Aliment Pharmacol Ther. 1993;7(3):247–57. Epub 1993/06/01.
82. Tonelli F, Fratini G, Nesi G, Tommasi MS, Batignani G, Falchetti A, et al. Pancreatectomy in multiple endocrine neoplasia type 1-related gastrinomas and pancreatic endocrine neoplasias. Ann Surg. 2006;244(1):61–70. Epub 2006/06/24.
83. Lopez CL, Waldmann J, Fendrich V, Langer P, Kann PH, Bartsch DK. Long-term results of surgery for pancreatic neuroendocrine neoplasms in patients with MEN1. Langenbecks Arch Surg. 2011;396(8):1187–96. Epub 2011/08/02.
84. Cadiot G, Vuagnat A, Doukhan I, Murat A, Bonnaud G, Delemer B, et al. Prognostic factors in patients with Zollinger-Ellison syndrome and multiple endocrine neoplasia type 1. Groupe d'Etude des Neoplasies Endocriniennes Multiples (GENEM and groupe de Recherche et d'Etude du Syndrome de Zollinger-Ellison (GRESZE)). Gastroenterology. 1999;116(2):286–93.
85. Fraker DL, Norton JA. The role of surgery in the management of islet cell tumors. Gastroenterol Clin North Am. 1989;18(4):805–30. Epub 1989/12/01.
86. Melvin WS, Johnson JA, Sparks J, Innes JT, Ellison EC. Long-term prognosis of Zollinger-Ellison syndrome in multiple endocrine neoplasia. Surgery. 1993;114(6):1183–8. Epub 1993/12/01.
87. Stabile BE, Passaro Jr E. Benign and malignant gastrinoma. Am J Surg. 1985;149(1):144–50. Epub 1985/01/01.
88. MacFarlane MP, Fraker DL, Alexander HR, Norton JA, Lubensky I, Jensen RT. Prospective study of surgical resection of duodenal and pancreatic gastrinomas in multiple endocrine neoplasia type 1. Surgery. 1995;118(6):973–9. discussion 9-80. Epub 1995/12/01.
89. Veldhuis JD, Norton JA, Wells Jr SA, Vinik AI, Perry RR. Surgical versus medical management of multiple endocrine neoplasia (MEN) type I. J Clin Endocrinol Metab. 1997;82(2):357–64. Epub 1997/02/01.
90. Malagelada JR, Edis AJ, Adson MA, van Heerden JA, Go VL. Medical and surgical options in the management of patients with gastrinoma. Gastroenterology. 1983;84(6):1524–32. Epub 1983/06/01.
91. Mignon M, Cadiot G. Diagnostic and therapeutic criteria in patients with Zollinger-Ellison syndrome and multiple endocrine neoplasia type 1. J Intern Med. 1998;243(6):489–94. Epub 1998/07/29.
92. Mignon M. Diagnostic and therapeutic strategies in Zollinger-Ellison syndrome associated with multiple endocrine neoplasia type I (MEN-I): experience of the Zollinger-Ellison Syndrome Research Group: Bichat 1958–1999. Bull Acad Natl Med. 2003;187(7):1249–58. discussion 59-60. Epub 2004/05/19.
93. Townsend Jr CM, Thompson JC. Gastrinoma. Semin Surg Oncol. 1990;6(2):91–7. Epub 1990/01/01.
94. Boudreaux JP, Putty B, Frey DJ, Woltering E, Anthony L, Daly I, et al. Surgical treatment of advanced-stage carcinoid tumors: lessons learned. Ann Surg. 2005;241(6):839–45. discussion 45-6. Epub 2005/05/25.
95. Arnold R, Wied M, Behr TH. Somatostatin analogues in the treatment of endocrine tumors of the gastrointestinal tract. Expert Opin Pharmacother. 2002;3(6):643–56. Epub 2002/12/11.
96. Shojamanesh H, Gibril F, Louie A, Ojeaburu JV, Bashir S, Abou-Saif A, et al. Prospective study of the antitumor efficacy of long-term octreotide treatment in patients with progressive metastatic gastrinoma. Cancer. 2002;94(2):331–43. Epub 2002/03/20.

97. Rinke A, Muller HH, Schade-Brittinger C, Klose KJ, Barth P, Wied M, et al. Placebo-controlled, double-blind, prospective, randomized study on the effect of octreotide LAR in the control of tumor growth in patients with metastatic neuroendocrine midgut tumors: a report from the PROMID Study Group. J Clin Oncol. 2009;27(28):4656–63. Epub 2009/08/26.
98. Wymenga AN, Eriksson B, Salmela PI, Jacobsen MB, Van Cutsem EJ, Fiasse RH, et al. Efficacy and safety of prolonged-release lanreotide in patients with gastrointestinal neuroendocrine tumors and hormone-related symptoms. J Clin Oncol. 1999;17(4):1111. Epub 1999/11/24.
99. Yao JC, Phan AT, Chang DZ, Wolff RA, Hess K, Gupta S, et al. Efficacy of RAD001 (everolimus) and octreotide LAR in advanced low- to intermediate-grade neuroendocrine tumors: results of a phase II study. J Clin Oncol. 2008;26(26):4311–8. Epub 2008/09/10.
100. Yao JC, Shah MH, Ito T, Bohas CL, Wolin EM, Van Cutsem E, et al. Everolimus for advanced pancreatic neuroendocrine tumors. N Engl J Med. 2011;364(6):514–23. Epub 2011/02/11.
101. Raymond E, Dahan L, Raoul JL, Bang YJ, Borbath I, Lombard-Bohas C, et al. Sunitinib malate for the treatment of pancreatic neuroendocrine tumors. N Engl J Med. 2011;364(6): 501–13. Epub 2011/02/11.
102. Strosberg JR, Fine RL, Choi J, Nasir A, Coppola D, Chen DT, et al. First-line chemotherapy with capecitabine and temozolomide in patients with metastatic pancreatic endocrine carcinomas. Cancer. 2011;117(2):268–75. Epub 2010/09/09.
103. Kwekkeboom D, Krenning EP, de Jong M. Peptide receptor imaging and therapy. J Nucl Med. 2000;41(10):1704–13. Epub 2000/10/19.

Chapter 5
Clinical Manifestations of Multiple Endocrine Neoplasia, Type 1

Susan Yuditskaya and Monica C. Skarulis

Multiple endocrine neoplasia type 1 (MEN1) is an autosomal dominant condition that results from inactivating mutations of the MEN1 gene (11q13) encoding *menin*, a tumor suppressor protein whose biochemical function has not yet been fully characterized. There are few hereditary cancer syndromes that can compare with the challenges associated with MEN1. Patients manifest clinically important, classical tumors (parathyroid, enteropancreatic, and pituitary) over many decades, often starting in young adulthood and occasionally in early childhood. These manifestations require expert medical and surgical interventions to arrest or ameliorate metabolic and neoplastic complications. Despite its high penetrance (95–100 % by age 60), MEN1 is a disease of considerable phenotypic heterogeneity. A few kindreds with distinctive phenotypic manifestations have been found; however, no consistent genotype–phenotype correlations have been identified. Pathologic mutations are found throughout the MEN1 gene locus and no particular mutation hotspots have surfaced among over 1,000 known germline MEN1 mutations [1]. The lack of known hotspots has implications in genetic testing of probands; the entire MEN1 gene sequence must be analyzed. Furthermore, in about 10–30 % of MEN1 kindreds and in 35–50 % of sporadic cases, no mutation is detectable by sequencing of the coding regions of the MEN1 gene, as can happen for instance with whole gene deletions, or in cases of somatic mosaicism [2–5]. These limitations have impeded efforts to establish genotype–phenotype correlations.

The phenotypic heterogeneity inherent in MEN1 can be explained, in part, by Knudson's two-hit hypothesis [6]. The germline MEN1 mutation, present in all diploid cells of the body, is usually inherited in heterozygous form. A tumor is subsequently generated only when the MEN1 locus of the normal allele suffers a mutation

S. Yuditskaya, M.D. • M.C. Skarulis, M.D. (✉)
Diabetes, Endocrine, and Obesity Branch, National Institute of Diabetes, Digestive and Kidney Diseases, National Institutes of Health, 31 Center Drive, Bethesda, MD 20892, USA
e-mail: monicas@intra.niddk.nih.gov

J.R. Pisegna (ed.), *Management of Pancreatic Neuroendocrine Tumors*,
DOI 10.1007/978-1-4939-1798-3_5

at the somatic level, within a cell of a susceptible tissue. Indeed, genetic analysis of various tissue-origin tumors arising in the setting of MEN1 has shown loss of heterozygosity at the MEN1 locus. The second mutation is necessary for tumor development, and leads to diversity of organ involvement. It sets the timing and potentially alters the severity of the clinical presentation of the tumor, thus leading to heterogeneity, even among affected members of the same family. It should be noted, however, that the second hit promotes, but may not necessarily be sufficient, to induce tumorigenesis [7, 8].

The clinical presentations of MEN1-related tumors may also be modified by the nature of the second-hit mutation. For example, a large deletion or frameshift resulting in a nonfunctional menin product may manifest differently from a missense point mutation or small in-frame deletion in which some degree of menin protein function is retained [4]. These differences could potentially vary widely from person to person, from tissue to tissue, and even among tumors within the same tissue. There are also at least 24 known normal variant polymorphisms of the MEN1 gene [1, 5].

Inheritance of the MEN1 gene mutation confers a predisposition to tumorigenesis at a young age. MEN1-associated tumors have been found in affected children; the youngest reported case is a 5-year-old with a pituitary macroadenoma showing loss of MEN1 gene heterozygosity [9]. The most highly penetrant of the MEN1 endocrinopathies, primary hyperparathyroidism (PHPT) secondary to cellular hyperplasia/multiple adenomas, occurs in 90 % of MEN1 patients between age 20 and 25 [5], in contrast to age 40–50 in sporadic non-MEN1-associated PHPT. A similar pattern of younger age of onset for MEN1-associated tumors compared to sporadic tumors is noted for most but not all tumor types.

MEN1 is considered the most wide ranging of tumor syndromes, with the potential to affect 25 different tissue types [3]. Rodent studies of tissue-specific MEN1 knockout mutations have demonstrated that absence of menin does not affect all tissues; for instance, absence of the MEN1 gene in mouse hepatocytes caused no abnormality at all [3, 4, 10]. In tissues impacted by reduced menin activity or level, the clinical manifestations are the aggregate effects of four levels of multiplicity—multiple tissue types involved, cellular hyperplasia of an affected tissue, multiple scattered tumors arising from vulnerable cell types within a heterogeneous tissue, and multiple contiguous tumors with distinct clonal origins in a homogeneous tissue [11].

The clinical diagnosis of MEN1 is based on guidelines established in 2001 [12, 13]. In an individual lacking a clear family history, the diagnosis is based on the presence of at least two of the three classical MEN1-associated tumors, including parathyroid hyperplasia, enteropancreatic endocrine tumor, or pituitary adenoma. If an individual is a member of a known MEN1 family, the diagnosis is made once any one of these tumors arise. In 2012, the clinical practice guidelines were updated with the addition of genetic screening of first degree relatives of known pathologic MEN1 gene mutation carriers. The identification of mutation carriers targets them for routine biochemical and clinical surveillance starting prior to age 5 (Table 5.1). MEN1 gene testing is also recommended for individuals presenting with atypical findings, including multiple parathyroid adenomas prior to age 40, recurrent hyperparathyroidism, gastrinomas, multiple pancreatic neuroendocrine tumors, or two nonclassical MEN1-associated tumors [13].

Table 5.1 Suggested screening for clinical manifestations of MEN1

Tumor	Age to begin	Annual biochemistry	Imaging
Parathyroid	8	Ionized calcium, PTH	None
Gastrinoma	20	Gastrin—if high then gastric pH measurement	None
Insulinoma	5	Fasting glucose, insulin, proinsulin	None
Other GEP-NET	<10	Chromogranin-A, pancreatic polypeptide, glucagon, VIP	Annual SRS, CT or MRI
Pituitary	5	PRL, IGF-1	MRI every 3 years
Adrenal	<10	Only as dictated by signs & symptoms and/or tumor >1 cm	Annual MRI or CT
Foregut carcinoid	20	None	MRI or CT every 1–2 years

Modified from Thakker et al. JCEM 2012 (13)

In this chapter, we attempt to describe the wide breadth of clinical manifestations of this heterogeneous disease and discuss both classical and nonclassical tumors related to loss of the tumor suppressor protein, menin.

5.1 Classical Tumors

5.1.1 Parathyroid Neoplasia

PHPT is the most common abnormality in MEN1, affecting 90–100 % of MEN1 patients by age 50. The average age of onset is 20–25 years, and it is often the first endocrinopathy that manifests in MEN1 patients. The gender distribution is more balanced in MEN1-associated PHPT as compared to sporadic PHPT, which has a threefold female predominance. MEN1 parathyroids are asymmetrically enlarged with multiple monoclonal tumors, in contrast to sporadic disease, which typically involves a solitary parathyroid adenoma. Ectopic or supernumerary parathyroid tissue is found in areas predicted by embryological migration of the third and fourth pharyngeal pouch (retroesophageal, intrathyroidal, or intrathymic) in approximately 20–30 % of cases [14]. The tumors are generally benign; however, there have been several case reports of parathyroid carcinoma in the setting of MEN1, but their incidence appears to be similar to that in the general population [17].

A cross-sectional analysis of 469 patients with sporadic PHPT and 64 patients with MEN1-related PHPT showed similar degrees of hypercalcemia, urinary calcium excretion, and nephrolithiasis, but at lower parathyroid hormone (PTH) levels in those with MEN1 (113.8 pg/mL vs. 173 pg/mL). MEN1 patients under the age of 50 were more likely to have an inappropriately normal-range PTH level (38 % versus 6 % in sporadic PHPT) [15]. Interestingly, the study found that the combination of a "normal" PTH level in a patient less than 50 years old with clinical signs of hyperparathyroidism conferred a 13.5 times higher risk of being affected by MEN1.

By applying these criteria to a cohort of sporadic hyperparathyroidism patients, the authors identified an additional MEN1 patient confirmed by genetic testing.

Despite the milder degree of PTH aberration, adverse effects on bone mineral density appear to be more pronounced in MEN1-associated hyperparathyroidism than in sporadic PHPT. MEN1 patients with hyperparathyroidism often already have osteopenia in their 20s or 30s [15, 16], and the degree of bone mineral density loss is greater when compared to sporadic hyperparathyroidism [15]. This apparent vulnerability of the bone, coupled with the observation of significantly lower serum phosphate levels in the MEN1 patients compared to sporadic cases has led to speculation regarding enhanced PTH bioactivity or downregulation of the calcium sensing receptors in MEN1.

In contrast to sporadic PHPT, the most notable clinical characteristic of MEN1-associated hyperparathyroidism is its high recurrence rate. Among patients who achieved normocalcemia immediately following parathyroidectomy in the NIH series, approximately 40 % had recurrence of PHPT at 10 years, and it is expected that with longer observation, most if not all patients will eventually develop recurrence. Subtotal (3–3.5 glands) parathyroidectomy with cervical thymectomy is preferred to lesser operations (2.5 glands removed or less) for long-term remission, and total parathyroidectomy is associated with high rates of hypoparathyroidism despite immediate autograft. Approaches differ among institutions as do cure rates, recurrence rates, and complications [18–22]. Subtotal parathyroidectomy versus total parathyroidectomy with autograft reimplantation of the most normal appearing parathyroid immediately or after cryopreservation [23] is still debated.

It is possible that the coexistence of other MEN1-related tumors may influence the course of PHPT and its response to surgical therapy. Coexistent Zollinger-Ellison syndrome is reported by Norton et al. to be associated with more clinically aggressive PHPT, nephrolithiasis, and higher persistent disease and recurrence rates following surgical management of the hyperparathyroidism over a 16-year follow-up period. It was noted that the biochemical parameters of Zollinger-Ellison syndrome also improved with correction of hypercalcemia [24].

In light of the high recurrence rate of MEN1-associated hyperparathyroidism, even with resection of more than three glands, long-term screening for recurrence following curative surgery is important.

5.1.2 Neuroendocrine Enteropancreatic Tumors

Neuroendocrine enteropancreatic tumors (NETs) are often multiple (Fig. 5.1), and can originate from the pancreas or arise in the duodenum, a common location for gastrinomas (>80 %) and rare tumors, such as somatostatinomas (44 %) and VIPomas (10 %). The penetrance of pancreatic neuroendocrine tumors as a phenotypic trait of MEN1, collectively, is second only to parathyroid neoplasia, and approaches 80–90 % by 60 years of age. Parathyroid disease typically manifests earlier than NET, and like parathyroid tumors, NETs arise at least a decade earlier

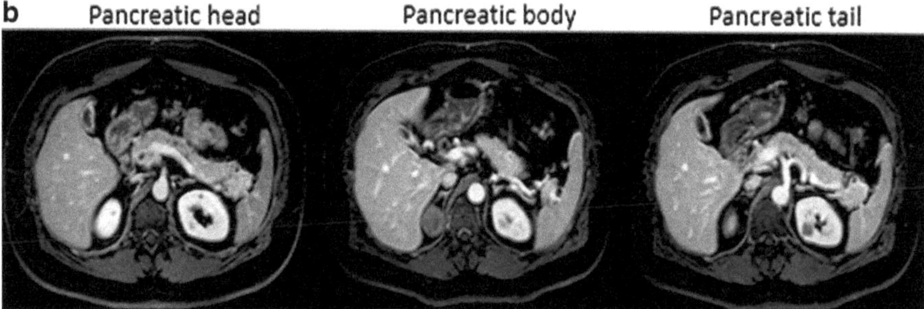

Fig. 5.1 Octreotide scan showing foci of uptake in the head, body, and tail of the pancreas (**a**) in a 43-year-old man with MEN1, corresponding to rim-enhancing pancreatic neuroendocrine tumors on MRI post-contrast images (**b**)

than in the case of sporadic NET. Loss of 11q13 heterozygosity was demonstrated in MEN1-related insulinoma in 1988 [25], pancreatic ductal/acinar cells, the putative precursor pancreatic islet tumors in 2004 [26], and duodenal gastrin- and somatostatin-secreting NET in 2007 [27]. Multifocal tumors within the same individual often demonstrate different 11q13 deletion patterns, implying distinct clonal origins.

5.1.2.1 Nonfunctioning Neuroendocrine Enteropancreatic Tumors

Nonfunctioning NETs affect 60–100 % of patients with MEN1, and primarily occur in the pancreas itself. These tumors do not secrete bioactive substances or hormones that lead to clinical symptoms, but express somatostatin receptor (SST) isoforms, in particular the high affinity SST2 [28], and are positive on immunohistochemical stain for various hormones. Although asymptomatic until they are large enough to cause obstruction or mass effect, the nonfunctioning pancreatic neuroendocrine tumors have a high malignancy rate estimated at 64–92 %. The risk of malignancy and the presence of liver metastases increase proportionally with the size of the tumor. Triponez et al. found liver metastases in 4 % of MEN1 patients with nonfunctional NET less than 1 cm in diameter, in 10 % with tumors 1.1–2 cm, in 18 % with tumors 2.1–3 cm, and in 43 % with tumors greater than 3 cm [29]. The French GTE cohort also documented a decreased survival rate in patients with nonfunctioning NET compared to those without NET. Surgical resection of nonfunctioning NET less than 2 cm in size does not improve recurrence, progression, or survival rates compared to those without NET [30]. These observations add to the notion that the larger sized NETs are responsible for the increased mortality rate noted among MEN1 patients with nonfunctioning NET [31]. A recent Japanese study of MEN1-associated nonfunctioning NET assessed imaging over a period of 2–10 years, confirming that patients with tumors less than 2 cm in size did not develop locoregional or liver metastases over the period of study, whereas the majority of patients with tumors greater than 3.5 cm in size showed disease progression with the appearance of additional NET (at times very fast-growing), and lymph nodes or liver metastases [32]. Overall, MEN1-associated nonfunctioning NETs tend to be smaller on average than those reported in sporadic cases (mean 4 cm [33]).

The incidence and prevalence of nonfunctioning neuroendocrine tumors have increased dramatically over the past three decades [28], presumably attributable to serum protein biomarker screening with chromogranin A and pancreatic polypeptide [34] and advances in imaging science. Detection rates of NET by CT or MRI are size dependent: less than 20 % of tumors less than 1 cm, 30–50 % of tumors between 1 cm and 3 cm, and greater than 70 % of tumors larger than 3 cm are successfully imaged [31, 35, 36]. Optimization of computerized tomography techniques, including rapid bolus contrast injection and scanning during the arterial phase using thin cross-sectional slices, has led to higher detection rates of small NET. Magnetic resonance imaging sequences to minimize motion artifact and use of algorithms for fat suppression improve detection. It may be argued that additional efforts to increase identification of smaller tumors may not lead to improvement in clinical outcomes; however, addressing technical challenges such as visualizing tumors with vascularity and tissue characteristics similar to surrounding non-neoplastic tissue, and filtering "noise" associated with thinner CT cross-sections will likely increase detection rates of tumors of all sizes.

The burgeoning field of functional and molecular imaging is increasingly more important for NET imaging [31, 37]. In addition to contributing to improved detection rates of tumors not readily visualized on conventional anatomical imaging, these studies offer metabolic or functional activity information about the tumors, which cannot be inferred from CT or MRI. The ubiquity of SST2 on nonfunctional NET cells has allowed somatostatin receptor scintigraphy (SRS) with radiolabeled octreotide to become a mainstay in determining NET status in MEN1 patients, and the procedure of choice for doing so [28, 38, 39]. Gallium-labeled somatostatin analog PET scanning has emerged as an important alternative to octreotide scans for NET detection, with better resolution than SRS done in tandem with CT [28, 40].

It should be mentioned that, although conventional transabdominal ultrasonography has low sensitivity for the detection of NET, endoscopic ultrasound is an extremely useful tool for imaging nonfunctional MEN1-associated NET, with a detection rate of 54–85 % [31]. The need for conscious sedation during this procedure limits its use as a first-line study for the detection of these tumors.

5.1.2.2 Gastrinoma

Gastrin-secreting tumors account for 50 % of all MEN1-related NET and usually manifest with clinical signs and symptoms of diarrhea, steatorrhea, and dyspepsia from hypersecretion of hydrochloric acid from hyperplastic parietal cells in the stomach and duodenum. Gastrinomas can arise in a variety of locations including the pancreas, lymphatic system, gallbladder, biliary tree, and stomach. However, the vast majority (80 %) occur in the duodenum as multiple small subcentimeter nodules in the duodenal submucosa. The majority of MEN1 gastrinomas coexist with other NET [41, 42].

As the tumor burden of gastrinoma increases, Zollinger-Ellison syndrome develops, leading to ulcerations in the stomach and duodenum, gastrointestinal bleeding, and ultimately perforation, if not treated. Approximately 80 % of MEN1 patients with gastrinomas have clinical Zollinger-Ellison syndrome. Prior to the use of high-dose histamine H2 receptor antagonists and the availability of proton-pump inhibitors, gastric and duodenal perforation related to Zollinger-Ellison syndrome was a major cause of morbidity and mortality in MEN1 patients [34]. Zollinger-Ellison syndrome is discussed in further detail elsewhere in this edition.

Interestingly, curative management of MEN1-related hyperparathyroidism is associated with amelioration of the clinical manifestations of coexisting hypergastrinemia. There is no apparent effect of the treatment of gastrinoma on the course of coexisting hyperparathyroidism [24, 43, 44].

5.1.2.3 Insulinoma

Tumors arising from the pancreatic β-cells occur in 21–30 % of MEN1 patients. One-third of MEN1 patients with insulinoma will have coexisting gastrinoma. The clinical manifestations in MEN1 vary slightly from sporadic insulinoma; however, the diagnostic approach (documentation of elevated insulin, proinsulin, and C-peptide levels during hypoglycemia) is the same. MEN1-associated insulinomas come to clinical attention approximately 10 years earlier than sporadic insulin secreting tumors, most prior to age 40, with many appearing prior to age 20 [45]. The majority of MEN1-associated insulinomas are less than 2 cm, have a low mitotic rate (Ki-67 < 2 %), and do not demonstrate angioinvasion or metastases.

During supervised fasting, MEN1 patients with insulinoma often fail to manifest neuroglycopenic symptoms during hypoglycemia, for unclear reasons [46]. Blunting or absence of typical adrenergic symptoms can lead to profound consequences, including hypoglycemic seizures, demyelinating sensory-motor polyneuropathy, or focal neuropathies, leading to the delay of the diagnosis. This point is exemplified by the case of a 17-year-old boy initially diagnosed with epilepsy, who eventually came to the diagnosis of MEN1 with the discovery of insulinoma-related hypoglycemia and hyperparathyroidism [47].

5.1.2.4 Glucagonoma and Other Rare NET

Tumors originating from pancreatic α-cells that secrete glucagon are reported in approximately 3 % of MEN1 patients. In contrast to insulinomas, the majority of glucagonomas are malignant and typically occur in the pancreatic tail. As in insulinoma, the clinical presentation is more subtle in MEN1 compared to the typical syndrome associated with sporadic glucagonomas, which consists of necrolytic migratory erythema, weight loss, anemia, and stomatitis. In MEN1, the only findings may be glucose intolerance and elevated circulating glucagon levels. The insidious nature and mild clinical manifestations may lead to delayed diagnosis. In fact, 50 % of MEN1 patients with glucagonoma present with metastatic disease at the time of diagnosis.

Enteropancreatic tumors secreting somatostatin or somatotropin (GHRH) are found in less than 1 % of MEN1 patients [48, 49]. In the case of somatostatinomas, 40 % are found in the duodenum or jejunum with signs and symptoms including cholelithiasis, steatorrhea, achlorhydria, and insulin resistance, but as with insulinomas and glucagonomas, the clinical presentation tends to be more insidious in MEN1 patients than in sporadic cases [50]. GHRHomas, manifesting with acromegaly, are found in the lungs (>50 %), pancreas (30 %), and small intestine (10 %) [50].

VIPomas (vasoactive intestinal polypeptidomas) have been reported in few patients with MEN1 [51], and can be recognized by the WDHA syndrome (watery diarrhea, hypokalemia, and achlorhydria) [52] and high plasma VIP levels. These tumors, like glucagonomas, predominantly localize to the pancreatic tail.

Collectively for these very rare NETs, prognosis is poor if metastatic with approximately 50 % of patients surviving at 10 years.

5.1.3 Pituitary Tumors

Anterior pituitary tumors are the third most common neoplasm among the classical MEN1 tumors. The rate of penetrance of pituitary adenoma is 30–40 %, and pituitary adenoma is the initial manifestation of MEN1 in approximately 15 % of cases. The mean age of onset is during the late fourth decade (similar to sporadic cases), although the age at the time of the discovery of adenomas is reported from 5 to 90 years. In contrast to most other MEN1-related neoplasms in which there is no sex predilection, there appears to be a female predominance with pituitary tumors.

A characterization of MEN1-specific versus sporadic pituitary adenomas was first done in 1987 by Scheithauer et al. [53] who found that MEN1 pituitary adenomas are more often functioning, with the majority secreting prolactin or growth hormone. Since then, a number of additional studies from large registries have demonstrated that MEN1 pituitary adenomas tend to be macroadenomas more often than in non-MEN1 patients, 85 % vs. 42 %, respectively [54]. In the MEN1 cohort studied at the NIH, some of the pituitary microadenomas were multifocal [55]. MEN1 pituitary adenomas are also noted to display more aggressive characteristics such as local tissue invasion and lower response to treatment [56–58]. The cause of the invasive nature of these tumors is unclear, but it has been postulated to be related to loss of the tumor suppressive function of *menin* as loss of heterozygosity of the MEN1 gene is rarely found in non-MEN1 pituitary tumors in which other gene mutations have been implicated (e.g., GNAS1) [59].

Apart from these features, clinical manifestations of MEN1-associated pituitary adenomas are largely reflective of the hormones they secrete, as well as any mass effect they may exert. The hormonal profile of MEN1-associated pituitary adenomas is actually similar to that of sporadic pituitary adenomas, characterized as largely prolactin-secreting (60 %) or somatotropinomas (25 %), the latter occurring more frequently in patients over the age of 40. ACTH-secreting tumors leading to Cushing's disease (5 %), nonfunctioning or glycoprotein subunit secreting adenomas (5 %), and rare thyrotropinomas are also seen at lower rates. In addition, plurihormonal expression is observed more frequently in MEN1 pituitary adenomas, with prolactin and growth hormone being the most commonly co-secreted hormones.

A variant of the MEN1 phenotype has been observed in three large kindreds, in which the prevalence of prolactinoma is much higher than in the typical MEN1 population (40 % vs. 22 %, respectively), while the prevalence of gastrinomas is much lower (10 % vs. 22 %) [60]. While each of the three kindreds has a different MEN1 gene mutation, it has been proposed that there may be a shared polymorphism tightly linked to the MEN1 gene that affects the clinical manifestation of the MEN1 disease [11, 25]. One of these kindreds is located on the Burin Peninsula of Newfoundland, and consists of four families sharing one common founder MEN1 mutation, named MEN1Burin, with a shared haplotype flanking the gene. The pituitary adenomas in this variant occur uniquely as prolactinomas, and symptoms on average manifest early in the third decade of life [60]. The other two kindreds originate from the East and West coast of the United States [11]. The caveat in diagnosis of this variant is that this pattern only becomes apparent in very large, well-studied cohorts.

5.2 Nonclassical Tumors

5.2.1 Non-pituitary Central Nervous System Tumors

Among 74 patients with MEN1 followed at the NIH with available brain imaging, the prevalence of intracranial meningioma was found to be 8 % [61]. MEN1-associated meningiomas were noted to occur as solitary tumors, to be hormonally inactive, and to be slow growing. The average tumor size in this series was 1.6 cm and the largest was 3 cm. Genetic analysis of a meningioma that required resection on clinical grounds confirmed loss of heterozygosity at the MEN1 gene locus.

Meningiomas are a late manifestation in the setting of MEN1, generally appearing in the fifth decade, raising the question whether the pathogenesis of this tumor is modified by the hormonal milieu or treatments administered over the course of MEN1. Interestingly, patients with meningioma are more likely to have Zollinger-Ellison syndrome [61]. This relationship is potentially supported by in vitro evidence that meningiomas may express cholecystokinin, neurotensin, and gastrin receptors, and that growth of ex vivo meningioma tissue cultures can be potentiated by gastrin. The association remains unclear, as there is no relationship between the magnitude of the plasma gastrin elevation and the presence of meningioma or the size of the tumor. It has also been postulated that prior cranial irradiation for treatment of invasive pituitary adenoma may promote the growth of meningiomas, a relationship well established among sporadic meningiomas [62, 63]. This causality has not been fully studied in MEN1; however, some meningiomas have occurred in patients who have not been exposed to radiation therapy [61].

Spinal ependymomas and schwannomas have also been reported in MEN1 patients [64], but loss of MEN1 gene heterozygosity has not yet been demonstrated for these tumors.

5.2.2 Carcinoid

Approximately 14 % of MEN1 patients develop carcinoid neuroendocrine tumor. In 1987, Duh et al. published a meta-analysis characterizing MEN-associated carcinoid tumors, which arise primarily from the foregut particularly the thymus, bronchi and gastric ECL cells. In contrast, sporadic carcinoid typically is found in the mid- and hind-gut [65].

Thymic carcinoid tumors have been recognized as part of the MEN1 syndrome since 1972 (Fig. 5.2) [66]. The risk of thymic carcinoid appears to be particularly high among male smokers [67]. Despite the overall rare occurrence, there is heightened concern to diagnose thymic carcinoid as early as possible due to the high rate of malignancy (80 %) and highly aggressive nature. These tumors are often clinically silent until local tissue invasion and metastases are extensive enough to cause a life-threatening situation, such as airway compromise or compression of the great vessels (e.g., SVC syndrome). Prognosis is poor, even if the patient is asymptomatic at the time of diagnosis, and despite radical surgical resection [68]. Thymic carcinoid, despite its rarity, is a significant cause of mortality among patients with MEN1 [69], especially as the more biochemically and clinically active causes of morbidity and mortality are being caught in their early stages and treated effectively. Because of the potentially disastrous implications of a clinically silent thymic carcinoid tumor, prophylactic thymectomy at the time of parathyroid surgery has been proposed [65, 67]. Detailed imaging of the chest and mediastinum with CT, MRI, and octreotide scanning are also strongly recommended as part of surveillance evaluation, largely for this reason [68].

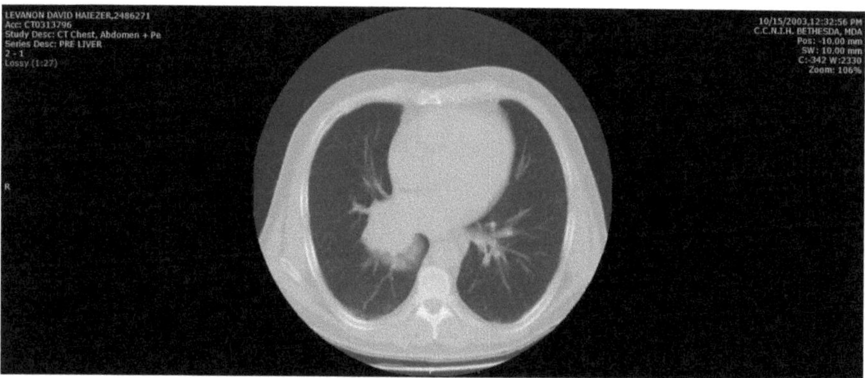

Fig. 5.2 CT-chest of a 54-year-old man with MEN1 showing a 10 cm lobulated bronchial carcinoid arising from the subcarinal space extending into the right hilum and thorax and invading the mediastinum and left atrial wall. The patient underwent resection of the right hilar mass with right pneumonectomy and left atrial reconstruction

In contrast to thymic carcinoids, bronchial carcinoid tumors occur more frequently in women; the majority (74 %) are benign and may be associated with the occurrence of pituitary adenomas. Typically multicentric, bronchial carcinoids develop synchronously or metasynchronously, a fact that may impact the aggressiveness of surgical management. The clinical course, however, tends to be indolent, although manifestations can be serious, including bronchial obstruction and other local mass effects [70].

The third type of MEN1-associated carcinoid arises from the gastric enterochromaffin-like (ECL) cells. These carcinoids develop under the condition of chronic gastrin excess, and in MEN1, occur almost entirely within the context of the Zollinger-Ellison syndrome (type 2 gastric carcinoid). Gastrin is mitogenic to ECL cells, and continuous exposure leads to hyperplastic proliferation and dysplastic changes which are precursors to gastric carcinoid tumor formation. MEN1-associated ECL cell carcinoid tumors have a malignancy rate of 10–30 % [71], and are usually multiple in number and small in size. There is no male or female predominance reported. ECL carcinoids are usually well differentiated but occasionally demonstrate locoregional extension. Endoscopic biopsy is regarded as the diagnostic method of choice for lesions less than 1 cm in size; endoscopic ultrasound is recommended for larger lesions to evaluate extent of invasion and facilitates fine-needle aspiration of submucosal lesions. Prognosis is linked to the course of the associated gastrinoma(s), but is generally good with an estimated 5-year survival of 62–75 % [72].

Loss of heterozygosity at the MEN1 gene locus 11q13 has been found in all type 2 gastric carcinoids. Interestingly, MEN1 gene LOH is also present in 17–73 % of type 1 gastric carcinoids (associated with hypergastrinemia related to achlorhydria/atrophic gastritis) and in 25–50 % of type 3 gastric carcinoids (unrelated to hypergastrinemia, and frequently malignant), although these do not develop in MEN1 patients.

Generally, MEN1-associated carcinoids are biochemically and clinically inactive, which contributes to their insidiousness. They are generally not associated with the typical bouts of flushing and bronchospastic dyspnea, although these signs can appear once the carcinoid metastasizes to the liver [73]. Foregut carcinoids secrete 5-hydroxytryptophan, but typically lack 5-HTP decarboxylase that converts 5-HTP to serotonin, and thus produce little to no serotonin [74]; along these lines, foregut carcinoids may not generate an elevated urinary 5-HIAA. Urinary serotonin, however, can be elevated, as 5-HTP decarboxylase is present in the kidney.

Exceptions to the rule that MEN1-associated foregut carcinoids are silent are well known to physicians who care for these patients. A case of WDHA syndrome was reported in an MEN1 patient with hyperparathyroidism and amenorrhea–galactorrhea syndrome that was attributed to a 370 g pancreatic carcinoid tumor secreting serotonin. Symptoms resolved following resection of the mass. Immunohistochemical staining of the tumor was positive only for serotonin, and was negative for vasoactive intestinal polypeptide, pancreatic polypeptide, glucagon, insulin, cholecystokinin, gastrin, and calcitonin. Diarrhea was attributed to serotonin excess [75].

Sporadic thymic carcinoids are known to be the source of ectopically secreted ACTH leading to Cushing's Syndrome, and has been reported in MEN1 [76]. Based on the above epidemiologic phenomena, it has been suggested that an ectopic ACTH syndrome occurring in the setting of MEN1 should arouse suspicion for bronchial carcinoid in women, and thymic carcinoid in men [65].

Of note, a large metastatic carcinoid burden can manifest with tryptophan deficiency, because of the conversion of tryptophan to 5-HTP by the tumor tissue. Signs of tryptophan deficiency can include decreased protein synthesis and pellagra due to depletion of nicotinic acid [77].

5.2.3 Adrenal Tumors

Adrenocortical neoplastic disease of one or both glands affects approximately 40 % of MEN1 patients [78] and can manifest as adenomas, hyperplasia, or adrenocortical carcinoma [5, 50, 79]. In most cases, MEN1-associated adrenal tumors are not hormonally active and benign, but both benign and malignant tumors can uncommonly be a source of adrenal Cushing's syndrome [80]. In a cohort of 400 patients with MEN1 evaluated at the NIH, three patients had ACTH-independent Cushing's syndrome attributable to adrenocortical pathology [55]. Albeit rarely, primary hyperaldosteronism has also been seen [81, 82]. It has been suggested that adrenocortical tumors larger than 3 cm possess higher malignant potential and should be resected [83].

Pheochromocytoma is exceedingly rare in MEN1, occurring in less than 1 % of patients [42, 84]. Only a few case reports exist, and all are unilateral. Genetic analysis of tumor tissue, as with the other MEN1 neoplasms, shows loss of MEN1 gene heterozygosity [85].

5.2.4 Smooth Muscle Tumors

Various kinds of leiomyomas, at times multicentric, are found in MEN1 patients, including esophageal smooth muscle [86], uterus, lung, and rectum [87]. A case report of a ureteral leiomyoma causing obstructive nephropathy [88] and a pulmonary leiomyoma arising from the lymphangitic smooth muscle have been reported [89]. Bladder, esophageal, and uterine leiomyomas were identified in a 50-year-old Korean woman with newly diagnosed MEN1 in 2008 [90].

Esophageal leiomyomas have a 5 % prevalence in MEN1, and uterine leiomyomas are estimated to affect about 30 % of women with MEN1 [11]. Loss of heterozygosity at the MEN1 locus has been proven in esophageal leiomyomata [91, 92] and uterine leiomyomas [92] excised from MEN1 patients, but not in sporadic smooth muscle tumors.

At our institution, a case of uterine leiomyosarcoma was identified in a 38-year-old woman with MEN1, progressive menorrhagia, and pelvic mass. Surgical resection of the mass showed a myxoid leiomyosarcoma of the uterus weighing 1.1 kg. The patient's menorrhagia was cured after resection of the mass, with no recurrence after 10 years of follow-up.

5.2.5 Cutaneous Manifestations

Lipomas, benign adipose tumors, were the first skin lesions to be recognized in association with MEN1 [93], and have a prevalence of approximately 30 % [85]. The majority appear subcutaneously on the trunk or extremities, but they also occur in viscera as there is an increased incidence of renal angiomyolipomas observed in MEN1 [91].

In 1997, the NIH MEN1 cohort was first recognized to have a high prevalence of angiofibromas (telangiectatic connective tissue papules), approaching 90 % (Fig. 5.3) [94]. Angiofibromas were previously believed to be pathognomonic for tuberous sclerosis. MEN1-associated angiofibromas are permanent acneiform

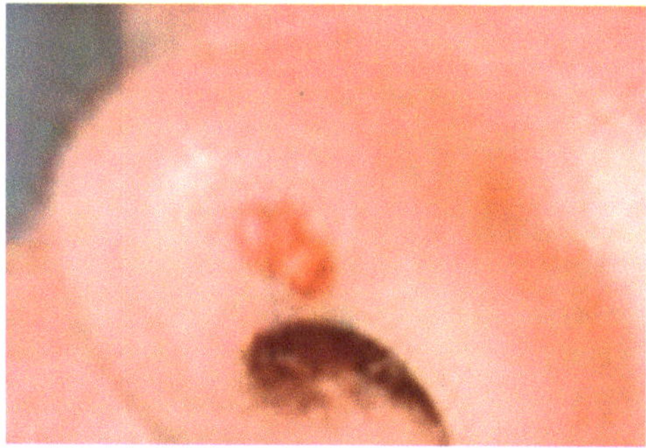

Fig. 5.3 Nasal angiofibroma

lesions that develop on the face, and in contrast to tuberous sclerosis, occur around the upper lip and vermilion border, and are smaller in size. In both diseases, however, angiofibromas demonstrate an identical histopathologic composition, consisting of dermal fibrosis with stellate fibroblasts and telangiectasias [94]. MEN1-associated angiofibromas were shown to have loss of MEN1 gene heterozygosity in perivascular cells [95].

Additionally, collagenomas (skin-colored papules consisting of collagen deposits in the reticular dermal layer) appear with significant frequency in MEN1 patients (70 % prevalence [85]), and are typically distributed over the upper torso neck and shoulders ranging in size from a few millimeters to a few centimeters. Of note, greater numbers of both angiofibromas and collagenomas occur with increasing age.

The diagnosis of MEN1 was made with 75 % sensitivity and 95 % specificity when the criteria of the presence of one or more collagenomas and three or more angiofibromas was applied to 110 consecutive patients with gastrinomas but unknown MEN1 status [96]. Because of their high prevalence, identification of cutaneous collagenomas and facial angiofibromas should raise suspicions for the diagnosis of MEN1 prior to manifestation of symptomatic disease [85].

Gingival papules, typically seen in tuberous sclerosis and Cowden's syndrome, are infrequent but have been reported in a few MEN1 patients [94].

In addition to these benign skin tumors, malignant melanoma has arisen in a few MEN1 kindreds; melanoma tumor tissue in these cases has not been assessed for loss of heterozygosity [97].

5.2.6 MEN1-Like Syndrome

About 30 % of patients with an MEN1-like phenotype have no identifiable MEN1 gene mutation. Failure to detect a mutation may be a result of methodology (failure to detect a deletion during amplification by polymerase chain reaction or a mutation in regulatory or untranslated regions). Serendipitously, a multi-tumor syndrome of overlapping MEN1 and MEN2 features that arose sporadically in rats led to the identification of another candidate gene. Affected rats were found to be homozygous for a tandem duplication of eight nucleotides in exon 2 of the *Cdkn1b* gene, which resulted in a frameshift and very low to absent expression of the p27 tumor suppressor protein in a variety of tissues. Affected animals had multifocal pituitary adenomas, bilateral adrenal and extra-adrenal pheochromocytomas, and hyperplasia of parathyroid tissue, pancreatic islet cells, and thyroid C-cells.

Since this discovery, *Cdkn1b* mutations have also been identified in several human cohorts of MEN1-like syndromes (Table 5.2). In 2009, Agarwal et al. screened 169 index cases of MEN1 without an identifiable MEN1 gene mutation for mutations in any of the seven CDKN1 genes [98]. Probable pathologic mutations in CDKN1 genes encoding p27, p21, p18, and p15 were found in just seven of these patients. Among them, there was not a characteristic constellation of manifestations

Table 5.2 Summary of probable pathogenic CDKI mutations associated with MEN1-like syndromes

Gene	Mutation	Protein	Index Case MEN1-like syndrome	Affected relatives	Reference
Cdkn1b	W76X	p27	GH-secreting pituitary adenoma + 1°HPT	Sister w/mutation & renal angiomyolipoma	[99]
Cdkn1b	K25fs	p27	Small-cell neuroendocrine cervical carcinoma, ACTH-secreting pituitary adenoma, 1°HPT	None known	[100]
Cdkn1b	ATG-7 (g>c)	p27	1°HPT (1 parathyroid tumor), stomach problems, bilateral nonfunctioning adrenal masses, uterine fibroids	2 asymptomatic daughters	[98]
Cdkn1b	P95S	p27	1°HPT (2 parathyroid tumors), ZES, masses in duodenum and tail of pancreas	None known	[98]
Cdkn1b	Stop>Q	p27	1°HPT (3 parathyroid tumors)	Identical twin w/mutation & 1°HPT	[98]
Cdkn1a	N41D	p15	1°HPT (3 parathyroid tumors), skin schwannoma, meningioma, liver, hemangioma	None known	[98]
Cdkn1a	L64R	p15	1°HPT (3 parathyroid tumors), ZES, adrenal mass, prostate cancer	None known	[98]
Cdkn1b	V31L	p18	1°HPT (2 parathyroid tumors), breast cancer	Mother with 1°HPT, mutation status unknown	[98]
Cdkn1a	R67L	p21	1°HPT, macroprolactinoma	Sister w/mutation & 1°HPT + macroprolactinoma; mother w/1°HPT, mutation status unknown	[98]
Cdkn1b	P69L	p27	Multifocal bronchial carcinoid, primary hyperparathyroidism, nonfunctioning pituitary microadenoma, papillary thyroid carcinoma	None known	[101]

that distinguished the MEN1 syndrome related these mutations versus MEN1 gene mutations. CDKN1-associated MEN1 syndrome appears to be extremely rare (1.6 % of all tested cases).

5.3 Conclusion

The initial description of Wermer's syndrome in 1954 of a genetically transmitted condition of parathyroid, pancreatic, and pituitary tumors (the three "Ps") has evolved with recognition of the clinical manifestations arising from loss of *menin* tumor suppressor function in humans. The challenge of caring for a patient with MEN1 stems from striking a balance between preventing complications from advanced, unrecognized disease and performing risky unnecessary interventions before there is ample clinical indication. Multinational consortiums are needed to continue study of this rare disorder and frequent revision of guidelines to diagnose and treat these patients over their lifetime is critical as our knowledge of *menin-related* disease and other overlapping-related genetic syndromes advance.

References

1. Lemos MC, Thakker RV. Multiple endocrine neoplasia type 1 (MEN1): analysis of 1336 mutations reported in the first decade following identification of the gene. Hum Mutat. 2007;29(1):22–32.
2. Klein RD, et al. Clinical testing for multiple endocrine neoplasia type 1 in a DNA diagnostic laboratory. Genet Med. 2005;7(2):131–8.
3. Marx SJ. Molecular genetics of multiple endocrine neoplasia type 1 and type 2. Nat Rev Cancer. 2005;5:367–75.
4. Tsukada T, Nagamura Y, Ohkura N. MEN1 gene and its mutations: basic and clinical implications. Cancer Sci. 2009;100(2):209–15.
5. Falchetti A, et al. Multiple endocrine neoplasia type 1 (MEN1): not only inherited endocrine tumors. Genet Med. 2009;11(12):825–35.
6. Knudson AG. Hereditary cancer: two hits revisited. J Cancer Res Clin Oncol. 1996;122:134–40.
7. Karges W, et al. Clinical and molecular diagnosis of multiple endocrine neoplasia type 1. Langenbecks Arch Surg. 2002;386:547–52.
8. Falchetti A, et al. Allelic loss in parathyroid tumors from individuals homozygous for multiple endocrine neoplasia type 1. J Clin Endocrinol Metab. 1997;82(7):2278–82.
9. Stratakis CA, et al. Pituitary macroadenoma in a 5-year-old: an early expression of multiple endocrine neoplasia type 1. J Clin Endocrinol Metab. 2000;85(12):4776–80.
10. Scacheri PC, et al. Homozygous loss of menin is well tolerated in liver, a tissue not affected in MEN1. Mamm Genome. 2004;15:872–7.
11. Agarwal SK, et al. The MEN1 gene and pituitary tumors. Horm Res. 2009;71 Suppl 2:131–8.
12. Brandi ML, et al. Guidelines for diagnosis and therapy of MEN type 1 and type 2. J Clin Endocrinol Metab. 2001;86(12):5658–71.
13. Thakker RV, et al. Clinical practice guildelines for multiple endocrine neoplasia type 1 (MEN1). J Clin Endocrinol Metab. 2012;97(9):2990–3011.

14. Nilubol N, et al. Preoperative localizing studies for initial parathyroidectomy in MEN1 syndrome: is there any benefit? World J Surg. 2012;36:1368–74.
15. Eller-Vainicher C, et al. Sporadic and MEN1-related primary hyperparathyroidism: differences in clinical expression and severity. J Bone Miner Res. 2009;24(8):1404–10.
16. Burgess JR, et al. Osteoporosis in multiple endocrine neoplasia type 1. Arch Surg. 1999;134:1119–23.
17. delPozo C, et al. Parathyroid carcinoma in multiple endocrine neoplasia type 1. Case report and review of the literature. Hormones. 2011;10(4):326–31.
18. Elaraj DM, et al. Results of initial operation for hyperparathyroidism in patients with multiple endocrine neoplasia type 1. Surgery. 2003;134:858–65.
19. Rizzoli R, Green III J, Marx SJ. Primary hyperparathyroidism in familial multiple endocrine neoplasia type I: long-term follow-up of serum calcium levels after parathyroidectomy. Am J Med. 1985;78:467–74.
20. Twigt BA, et al. Differences between sporadic and MEN-related primary hyperparathyroidism: clinical expression, preoperative workup, operative strategy and follow-up. Orphanet J Rare Dis. 2013;8:50.
21. Hellman P, et al. Primary and reoperative parathyroid operations in hyperparathyroidism of multiple endocrine neoplasia type 1. Surgery. 1998;124:993–9.
22. Salmeron MDB, et al. Causes and treatment of recurrent hyperparathyroidism after subtotal parathyroidectomy in the presence of multiple endocrine neoplasia 1. World J Surg. 2010;34:1325–31.
23. Feldman AL, et al. Results of heterotopic parathyroid autotransplantation: a 13 year experience. Surgery. 1999;126:1042–8.
24. Norton JA, et al. Prospective study of surgery for primary hyperparathyroidism (HPT) in multiple endocrine neoplasia-type1 (MEN1), and Zollinger-Wllison syndrome (ZES): long-term outcome of a more virulent form of HPT. Ann Surg. 2008;247(3):501–10.
25. Larsson C, et al. Multiple endocrine neoplasia type 1 gene maps to chromosome 11 and is lost in insulinoma. Nature. 1988;332:85–7.
26. Vortmeyer AO, et al. Non-islet origin of pancreatic islet cell tumors. J Clin Endocrinol Metab. 2004;89:1934–8.
27. Anlauf M, et al. Allelic deletion of the MEN1 gene in duodenal gastrin and somatostatin cell neoplasms and their precursor lesions. Gut. 2007;56:637–44.
28. Giandomenico V, et al. Improving the diagnosis and management of neuroendocrine tumors: utilizing new advances in biomarker and molecular imaging science. Neuroendocrinology. 2013;98:16–30.
29. Triponez F, et al. Epidemiology data on 108 MEN1 patients from the GTE with isolated nonfunctioning tumors of the pancreas. Ann Surg. 2006;245(2):265–72.
30. Triponez F, et al. Is surgery beneficial for MEN-1 patients with small (=2 cm), nonfunctioning pancreaticoduodenal endocrine tumor? An analysis of 65 patients from the GTE. World J Surg. 2006;30:654–62.
31. Jensen RT, et al. Inherited pancreatic endocrine tumor syndromes: advances in molecular pathogenesis, diagnosis, management, and controversies. Cancer. 2008;113 Suppl 7:1807–43.
32. Sakurai A, et al. Long-term follow-up of patients with multiple endocrine neoplasia type 1. Endocr J. 2008;54(2):295–302.
33. Gullo L, et al. Nonfunctioning pancreatic endocrine tumors: a multicenter clinical study. Am J Gastroenterol. 2003;98(11):2435–9.
34. Pannett AAJ, Thakker RV. Multiple endocrine neoplasia type 1. Endocr Relat Cancer. 1999;6:449–73.
35. Metz DC, Jensen RT. Gastrointestinal neuroendocrine tumors: pancreatic endocrine tumors. Gastroenterology. 2008;135(5):1469–92.
36. Rockall AG, Reznek RH. Imaging of neuroendocrine tumours (CT/MR/US). Best Pract Res Clin Endocrinol Metab. 2007;21(1):43–68.
37. Philips S, et al. Pancreatic endocrine neoplasms: a current update on genetis and imaging. Br J Radiol. 2012;85:682–96.

38. van der Lely AJ, et al. Octreoscan radioreceptor imaging. Endocrine. 2003;20:307–11.
39. Öberg K. Pancreatic endocrine tumors. Semin Oncol. 2010;37:594–618.
40. Velikyan I, et al. In vivo binding of [68Ga]-DOTATOC to somatostatin receptors in neuroendocrine tumours—impact of peptide mass. Nucl Med Biol. 2010;37:265–75.
41. Norton JA, et al. Surgery to cure the Zollinger-Ellison syndrome. N Engl J Med. 1999;341(9):635–44.
42. Piecha G, Chudek J, Wiecek A. Multiple endocrine neoplasia type 1. Eur J Intern Med. 2008;19:99–103.
43. Mai HD, Sanowski RA. Regression of duodenal gastrinomas in a patient with multiple endocrine neoplasia type 1 after parathyroidectomy. Gastrointest Endosc. 1992;38(6):706–8.
44. Tonelli F, et al. Pancreatic endocrine tumors in multiple endocrine neoplasia type 1 syndrome: review of the literature. Endocr Pract. 2011;17 Suppl 3:33–40.
45. Trump D, et al. Clinical studies of multiple endocrine neoplasia type 1 (MEN1). QJM. 1996;89(9):653–69.
46. Hirshberg B, et al. Forty-eight-hour fast: the diagnostic test for insulinoma. J Clin Endocrinol Metab. 2000;85(9):3222–6.
47. de Paiva AR, et al. Multiple endocrine neoplasia type 1 presenting as refractory epilepsy and polyneuropathy—a case report. J Neurol Sci. 2012;315:172–75.
48. Garby L, et al. Clinical characteristics and outcome of acromegaly induced by ectopic secretion of growth hormone releasing hormone (GHRH): a French nationwide series of 21 cases. J Clin Endocrinol Metab. 2012;97(6):2093–104.
49. Saleem TF, et al. Acromegaly caused by growth hormone releasing hormone (GHRH) secreting tumor in multiple endocrine neoplasia (MEN-1). W V Med J. 2012;108(2):26–30.
50. Thakker RV. Multiple endocrine neoplasia type 1. Endocrinol Metab Clin North Am. 2000;29(3):541–67.
51. Masulovic D, et al. Hepatobiliary and pancreatic: pancreatic VIPomas associated with multiple endocrine neoplasia type 1. J Gastroenterol Hepatol. 2012;27:619.
52. Marks IN, Bank S, Louw JH. Islet cell tumor of the pancreas with reversible watery diarrhea and achylorhydraia. Gastroenterology. 1967;52(4):695–708.
53. Scheithauer BW, et al. Pituitary adenomas of the multpile endocrine neoplasia type 1 syndrome. Semin Diagn Pathol. 1987;4:205–11.
54. Verges B, et al. Pituitary disease in MEN type 1 (MEN1): data from the France-Belgium MEN1 multicenter study. J Clin Endocrinol Metab. 2002;87:457–65.
55. Simonds WF, et al. Cushing's syndrome in multiple endocrine neoplasia type 1. Clin Endocrinol (Oxf). 2012;76:379–86.
56. Burgess JR, et al. Spectrum of pituitary disease in multiple endocrine neoplasia type 1 (MEN 1): clinical, biochemical, and radiological features of pituitary disease in a large MEN1 kindred. J Clin Endocrinol Metab. 1996;81:2642–6.
57. Burgess JR, et al. Prolactinomas in a large kindred with multiple endocrine neoplasia type 1: clinical features and inheritance pattern. J Clin Endocrinol Metab. 1996;81:1841–5.
58. Beckers A, et al. The treatment of sporadic versus MEN1-related pituitary adenomas. J Intern Med. 2003;253:599–605.
59. Marx SJ, Nieman LK. Aggressive pituitary tumors in MEN1: do they refute the two-hit model of tumorigenesis? J Clin Endocrinol Metab. 2002;87(2):453–6.
60. Hao W, et al. Multiple endocrine neoplasia type 1 variant with frequent prolactinoma and rare gastrinoma. J Clin Endocrinol Metab. 2004;89(8):3776–84.
61. Asgharian B, et al. Meningiomas may be a component tumor of multiple endocrine neoplasia type 1. Clin Cancer Res. 2004;10:869–80.
62. Waga S, Handa H. Radiation-induced meningioma: with review of literature. Surg Neurol. 1976;5:215–9.
63. Rubinstein AB, et al. Radiation-induced cerebral meningioma: a recognizable entity. J Neurosurg. 1984;61:966–71.
64. Kato H, Uchimura I, Morohoshi M. Multiple endocrine neoplasia type 1 associated with spinal ependymoma. Intern Med. 1996;35:285–9.

65. Duh Q-Y, et al. Carcinoids associated with multiple endocrine neoplasia syndromes. Am J Surg Pathol. 1987;154:142–8.
66. Rosai J, Higa E, Davie J. Mediastinal endocrine neoplasm in patients with multiple endocrine adenomatosis. A previously unrecognized association. Cancer. 1972;29:1075–83.
67. Ferolla P, et al. Thymic neuroendocrine carcinoma (carcinoid) in multiple endocrine neoplasia type 1 syndrome: the Italian series. J Clin Endocrinol Metab. 2005;90:2603–9.
68. Gibril F, et al. Prospective study of thymic carcinoids in patients with multiple endocrine neoplasia type 1. J Clin Endocrinol Metab. 2003;88:1066–81.
69. Wilkinson S, et al. Cause of death in multiple endocrine neoplasia type 1. Arch Surg. 1993;128:683–90.
70. Sachithanandan N, Harle RA, Burgess JR. Bronchopulmonary carcinoid in multiple endocrine neoplasia type 1. Cancer. 2005;103:509–15.
71. Berna MJ, et al. A prospective study of gastric carcinoids and enterochromaffin-like cell changes in multiple endocrine neoplasia type 1 and Zollinger-Ellison syndrome. J Clin Endocrinol Metab. 2008;93(5):1582–91.
72. Massironi S, et al. Gastric carcinoids: between underestimation and overtreatment. World J Gastroenterol. 2009;15(18):2177–83.
73. Bordi C, et al. Aggressive forms of gastric neuroendocrine tumors in multiple endocrine neoplasia type 1. Am J Surg Pathol. 1997;21:1075–82.
74. Feldman JM. Carcinoid tumors and syndrome. Semin Oncol. 1987;15(3):237–46.
75. Lee CH, et al. Carcinoid tumor of the pancrease causing the diarrheogenic syndrome: report of a case combined with multiple endocrine neoplasia, type 1. Surgery. 1986;99(1):123–9.
76. Ghazi AA, et al. Cushing syndrome secondary to a thymic carcinoid tumor due to multiple endocrine neoplasia type 1. Endocr Pract. 2011;17:e92–6.
77. Swain CP, Tavill AS, Neale G. Studies of tryptophan and albumin metabolism in a patient with carcinoid syndrome, pellagra, and hypoproteinemia. Gastroenterology. 1976;71(3):484–9.
78. Skogseid B, et al. Clinical and genetic features of adrenocortical lesions in multiple endocrine neoplasia type 1. J Clin Endocrinol Metab. 1992;75:76–81.
79. Griniatsos JE, et al. Bilateral adrenocortical carcinoma in a patient with multiple endocrine neoplasia type 1 (MEN1) and a novel mutation in the MEN1 gene. World J Surg Oncol. 2011;9:6.
80. Haase M, et al. A new mutation in the menin gene causes the multiple endocrine neoplasia type 1 syndrome with adrenocortical carcinoma. Endocrine. 2011;39:153–9.
81. Fertig A, Webley M, Lynn JA. Primary hyperparathyroidism in a patient with Conn's syndrome. Postgrad Med J. 1980;56:45–7.
82. Beckers A, et al. Aldosterone-secreting adrenal adenomas as part of multiple endocrine neoplasia type 1 (MEN1): loss of heterozygosity for polymorphic chromosome 11 deoxyribonucleic acid markers, including the MEN1 locus. J Clin Endocrinol Metab. 1992; 75(2):564–70.
83. Marini F, et al. Multiple endocrine neoplasia type 1. Orphanet J Rare Dis. 2006;1(38):1750–72.
84. Marx SJ, et al. Multiple endocrine neoplasia type 1: clinical and genetic features of the hereditary endocrine neoplasias. Recent Prog Horm Res. 1999;54:397–438.
85. Schussheim DH, et al. Multiple endocrine neoplasia type 1: new clinical and basic findings. Trends Endocrinol Metab. 2001;12(4):173–8.
86. Dong Q, et al. Loss of heterozygosity at 11q13: analysis of pituitary tumors, lung carcinoids, lipomas, and other uncommon tumors in subjects with familial multiple endocrine neoplasia type 1. J Clin Endocrinol Metab. 1997;82(5):1416–20.
87. Igaz P. MEN1 clinical background. In: Balogh K, Patocs A, editors. Super MEN1: pituitary parathyroid and pancreas. New York: Landes Bioscience & Springer Science+Business Media; 2009. p. 1–15.
88. Ikota H, et al. Ureteral leiomyoma causing hydronephrosis in type 1 multiple endocrine neoplasia. Pathol Int. 2004;54:457–9.

89. Carnevale V, et al. Pulmonary lymphangioleiomyoma in a patient with multiple endocrine neoplasia type 1. J Endocrinol Invest. 1997;20(5):282–5.
90. Choi H, et al. Multiple endocrine neoplasia type 1 with multiple leiomyomas linked to a novel mutation in the MEN1 gene. Yonsei Med J. 2008;49(4):655–61.
91. Vortmeyer AO, et al. Multiple endocrine neoplasia type 1: atypical presentation, clinical course, and genetic analysis of multiple tumors. Mod Pathol. 1999;12(9):919–24.
92. McKeeby JL, et al. Multiple leiomyomas of the esophagus, lung, and uterus in multiple endocrine neoplasia type 1. Am J Pathol. 2001;159:1121–7.
93. Ballard HS, Frame B, Hartsock RJ. Familial multiple endocrine adenoma-peptic ulcer complex. Medicine. 1964;43:481–516.
94. Darling TN, et al. Multiple facial angiofibromas and collagenomas in patients with multiple endocrine neoplasia type 1. Arch Dermatol. 1997;133:853–7.
95. Vortmeyer AO, et al. Perivascular cells harboring multiple endocrine neoplasia type 1 alterations are neoplastic cells in angiofibromas. Cancer Res. 1999;59:274–8.
96. Asgharian B, et al. Cutaneous tumors in patients with multiple endocrine neoplasm type 1 (MEN1) and gastrinomas: prospective study of frequency and development of criteria with high sensitivity and specificity for MEN1. J Clin Endocrinol Metab. 2004;89:5328–36.
97. Nord B, et al. Malignant melanoma in patients with multiple endocrine neoplasia type 1 and involvement of the MEN1 gene in sporadic melanoma. Int J Cancer. 2000;87:463–7.
98. Agarwal SK, Mateo CM, Marx SJ. Rare germline mutations in cyclin-dependent kinase inhibitor genes in multiple endocrine neoplasia type 1 and related states. J Clin Endocrinol Metab. 2009;94:1826–34.
99. Pellegata NS, et al. Germ-line mutations in p27kip1 cause a multiple endocrine neoplasia syndrome in rats and humans. Proc Natl Acad Sci. 2006;103(42):15558–63.
100. Georgitsi M, et al. Germline cdkn1b/p27kip1 mutation in multiple endocrine neoplasia. J Clin Endocrinol Metab. 2007;92(8):3321–5.
101. Molatore S, et al. A novel germline CDKN1B mutation causing multiple endocrine tumors: clinical, genetic and functional characterization. Hum Mutat. 2010;31(11):E1825–35.

Chapter 6
Gastric Carcinoids: Classification and Diagnosis

Kali Zhou and Wendy Ho

Abbreviations

5-HIAA	5-hydroxylindoleacetic acid
CAG	Chronic atrophic gastritis
CT	Computed tomography
ECL	Enterochromaffin-like
EMR	Endoscopic mucosal resection
EUS	Endoscopic ultrasound
GC	Gastric carcinoid
GEP-NET	Gastroenteropancreatic-neuroendocrine tumor
MEN1	Multiple endocrine neoplasia type 1
SRS	Somatostatin receptor scintigraphy
WHO	World Health Organization
ZES	Zollinger-Ellison syndrome

K. Zhou, M.D.
Department of Medicine, UCLA, 57 Westwood Plaza, Suite B7-111, Mailcode 742430, Los Angeles, CA 90095, USA
e-mail: kalizhou26@gmail.com

W. Ho, M.D., M.P.H. (✉)
Department of Medicine, Division of Digestive Diseases, UCLA, 100 UCLA Medical Plaza, Suite 303, Los Angeles, CA 90095, USA
e-mail: wwho@mednet.ucla.edu

J.R. Pisegna (ed.), *Management of Pancreatic Neuroendocrine Tumors*,
DOI 10.1007/978-1-4939-1798-3_6

6.1 Epidemiology

In 1923, Max Askanazy first reported the presence of carcinoid tumors arising from the stomach. Williams and Sandler in 1963 began to classify carcinoids according their embryologic site of origin: foregut, midgut, and hindgut. In 2004, the World Health Organization (WHO) proposed the term gastroenteropancreatic-neuroendocrine tumor (GEP-NET) to describe carcinoids of the gastrointestinal system. Subsequently in 2010, WHO updated its classification based on tumor site of origin [1]. Staging of the tumor can also be accomplished by the TNM system (see Table 6.1). GEP-NET and gastrointestinal carcinoid are now used interchangeably. In general practice, gastric carcinoid (GC) refers to a histologically well-differentiated, low-grade neuroendocrine tumor. For a long time, gastric carcinoids were thought to be fairly rare, comprising only 2 % of all carcinoid tumors and 1 % of all stomach neoplasms. However, incidence over the last 50 years has been rising and is now determined to be at least 4.1 % of all carcinoid tumors [2]. A large component of the rise in incidence is due to several extrinsic factors, including wider use of endoscopy, increasing surveillance of disease, and more routine biopsies [3]. Patients who develop gastric carcinoid are predominantly female (64.5 %) with higher incidence rates seen in the black and Asian populations and white females. In most cases, disease is local, but distant metastasis or regional spread is evident at the time of diagnosis in 10–30 %. Prognosis is good with an overall survival of 64.7 % over 5 years [2].

Gastric carcinoid is classified into three distinct subtypes with type I and II taking a more benign course associated with hypergastrinemia and type III rising sporadically with greater malignant potential. The differences between the three subtypes will be outlined below. The type of gastric carcinoid significantly impacts diagnosis, treatment, and survival.

6.2 Classification (see Table 6.2)

6.2.1 Type I

Type I gastric carcinoid is the most common of the three types, accounting for 65–80 % of all gastric carcinoids [4, 5]. This type is seen primarily in patients with type A chronic atrophic gastritis (CAG), with or without pernicious anemia. Approximately 5 % of patients with CAG will develop gastric carcinoid [3]. The incidence of carcinoid tumors in pernicious anemia is up to 10 % [6]. CAG is an inflammatory condition characterized by loss of gastric glandular structures. In CAG, loss of these glands leads to hypochlorhydria or achlorhydria, stimulating chronic hypergastrinemia and subsequent enterochromaffin-like (ECL) cell hyperplasia and eventually carcinoid formation [7]. Type I gastric carcinoid is most common in women between 40 and 60 years old, frequently found in asymptomatic patients, and often discovered on routine endoscopy. Lesions are localized to the

Table 6.1 American Joint Committee on Cancer Staging for NETs of the stomach small intestine, colon, and rectum

Stage 0	TiS	Stomach	Carcinoma in situ/dysplasia (tumor size less than 0.5 mm), confined to mucosa		N0: No regional lymph nodes metastasis	M0: No distant metastasis
Stage I	T1*	Stomach/Duodenum/ Jejunum/Ileum	Tumor invades lamina propria or submucosa and size 1 cm or less			
		Ampulla	Tumor 1 cm or less			
		Colon or rectum	T1	Tumor invades lamina propria or submucosa and size 2 cm or less		
			T1a	Tumor size less than 1 cm in greatest dimension		
			T1b	Tumor size 1–2 cm in greatest dimension		
Stage IIA	T2*	Stomach/Duodenum/ Jejunum/Ileum	Tumor invades muscularis propria or size greater than 1 cm			
		Ampulla	Tumor greater than 1 cm			
		Colon or rectum	Tumor invades muscularis propria or size more than 2 cm with invasion of lamina propria or submucosa			
Stage IIB	T3*	Stomach	Tumor penetrates subserosa			
		Duodenum/Ampulla/ Jejunum/Ileum	Tumor invades muscularis propria into subserosal tissue without penetration of overlying serosa (jejuna or ileal tumors) or invades pancreas or retroperitoneum (ampullary or duodenal tumors) or into non-peritonealized tissues			
		Colon or rectum	Tumor invades through muscularis propria into the subserosa, or into non-peritonealized pericolic or perirectal tissues			
Stage III A	T4*	Duodenum/Ampulla/ Jejunum/Ileum	Tumor invades visceral peritoneum (serosa) or other organs or adjacent structures			
		Colon or rectum	Tumor invades peritoneum or other organs			
Stage III B	Any T				N1: Regional lymph node metastasis	
Stage IV	Any T				Any N	M1: Distant metastasis

The original source for this material is the *AJCC Cancer Staging Handbook*. 7th ed. (2010) published by Springer Science and Business Media LLC, www.springerlink.com

Table 6.2 Comparison of three types of gastric carcinoid

	% of all GC	Gender	Age	Disease association	Endoscopic appearance	Location in stomach	Gastrin level
Type 1	65–80 %	Female > male	40–60	Chronic atrophic gastritis	Multiple, small	Body and fundus	High
Type 2	5–6 %	Female = male	45	MEN1/ Zollinger-Ellison Syndrome	Multiple, small	Body, fundus, antrum	High
Type 3	14–25 %	Male > Female	50	None	Solitary, large, ulcerated	Anywhere	Normal

atrophic oxyntic mucosa found in the body or fundus of the stomach, are typically multicentric, small (less than 2 cm), and polypoid. Histologically, this tumor is well-differentiated and built up in a trabecular to solid pattern. The proliferative activity is low with a Ki-67 index usually less than 2 %. Type I gastric carcinoid is generally noninvasive, with 27 % of tumors limited to the mucosa, 64 % to submucosa, and only 9 % crossing into muscularis propria. Lymph node metastasis is only detected in 2–9 % of patients and risk increases with tumor size. Patients with type I gastric carcinoid carry an excellent prognosis with life expectancy equal to that of the general population [4, 5].

6.2.2 *Type II*

The second type of gastric carcinoid is seen only in patients with the genetic condition multiple endocrine neoplasia type 1 (MEN1) with Zollinger-Ellison syndrome (ZES). Studies have shown that anywhere between 0 and 33 % of MEN1/ZES patients develop gastric carcinoid. MEN1 is an autosomal dominant disorder secondary to a mutation on chromosome 11q13 and is characterized by the constellation of hyperparathyroidism, pituitary tumors, and pancreatic islet cell tumors. In the subset of patients with ZES, pancreatic gastrin-secreting tumors create a state of hypergastrinemia that leads to carcinoid development [8]. Type II gastric carcinoid encompasses 5–6 % of all gastric carcinoids [5]. These tumors are multiple and small and are usually found in the body and fundus of the stomach. However, unlike type 1 GC, they can occasionally also be localized in the antrum [3]. Gender distribution is equal and mean age of diagnosis is 45 years. Histologic findings are of a trabecular pattern with a proliferation rate of less than 2 %. Type II gastric carcinoids are of intermediate malignant potential, with lymph node metastases present in 10–30 % of patients. The 5-year survival rate is lower than type I at 60–75 % [4, 5]. Risk factors for type II gastric carcinoid development in patients with MEN1/ZES include high fasting serum gastrin levels and long disease duration. Tumors typically develop after 15–20 years of disease.

6.2.3 Type III

Type III gastric carcinoids are sporadic lesions that are not gastrin dependent. They comprise 14–25 % of all gastric carcinoids. There is no known association with a particular disease, although some patients may have second cancers. Mean age of diagnosis is slightly older at 50 and they are more common in men. The tumor is usually solitary instead of multiple, can be seen in any part of the stomach, and can be ulcerated. They are larger with 70 % of lesions greater than 1 cm in size. The histologic pattern is both solid and trabecular, and the proliferation rate can exceed 2 %. Type III gastric carcinoid is much more likely to infiltrate the muscularis propria or be angioinvasive with a majority of patients showing metastases at presentation to regional lymph nodes and the liver. Likelihood of metastasis correlates with the size of the lesion. The 5-year survival in type III gastric carcinoid is less than 50 %, dropping to 21 % if metastases are present [4, 5].

6.3 Clinical Presentation

Gastric carcinoids are frequently found incidentally at the time of surgery or during routine endoscopic procedures. Tumors are often asymptomatic, particularly with type I and type II gastric carcinoids. If symptoms do occur, they may result from local tumor mass effect, tumor-related fibrosis, or secreted bioactive products. Patients can experience vague abdominal pain, vomiting, dyspepsia, anemia, or occult blood in stool. In rare instances, more commonly with type III, patients can present with gastrointestinal hemorrhage secondary to vascular abnormalities. Less than 5–10 % of patients develop either typical or atypical carcinoid syndrome. Typical carcinoid syndrome occurs in less than 10 % of patients and manifests as cutaneous flushing of the face, neck, and upper chest with gut hypermotility leading to diarrhea. The flushing of atypical carcinoid is more extreme, purplish, patchy, intensely pruritic, and localized to the trunk and upper extremities [1, 4, 5]. The flushing of both typical and atypical carcinoid syndrome lasts 10–30 minutes.

6.4 Mechanism

Type I and II gastric carcinoids are associated with hypergastrinemia. Food stimulates G cells in the antrum of the stomach to produce gastrin, which stimulates cholecystokinin (CCK)-2 receptors on ECL cells to secrete histamine, which then bind to H2 receptors on parietal cells, causing them to secrete acid. The acid secretion then triggers somatostatin release, which acts as a negative feedback mechanism to decrease the amount of gastrin produced. In patients with CAG, the presence of achlorhydria leads to excess secretion of gastrin and stimulation of ECL cell hyperplasia (see Fig. 6.1). A risk factor for gastric carcinoid in CAG is ECL cell dysplasia, which may represent a precursor lesion [7]. Similarly, in pernicious anemia,

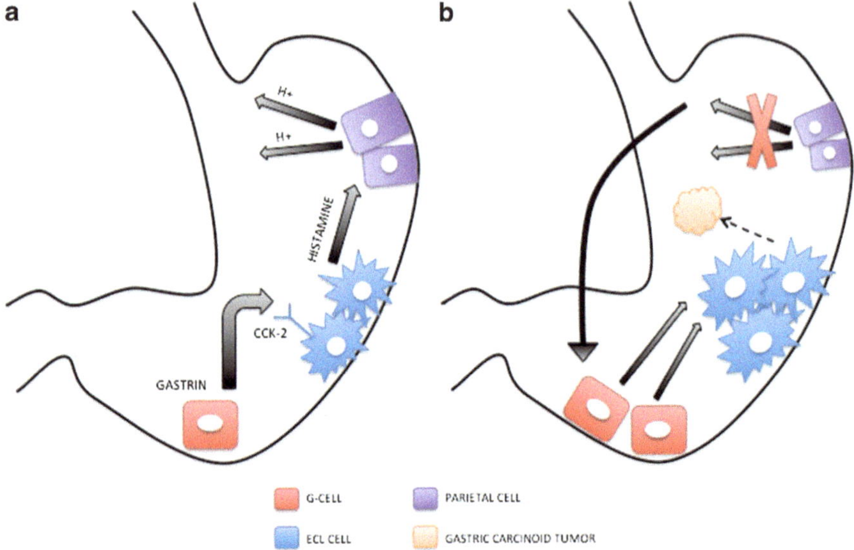

Fig. 6.1 Mechanism of gastrin stimulation in Type I gastric carcinoid. (**a**) G-cells in the antrum of the stomach secrete gastrin, which stimulates CCK-2 receptors on ECL cells to secrete histamine, which in turn causes acid secretion by parietal cells. (**b**) Achlorhydria secondary to parietal cell atrophy creates a feedback loop to G-cells, leading to excess gastrin production and ECL cell hyperplasia and subsequent transformation into type I gastric carcinoid

inflammation destroys parietal cells and decreases gastric acid secretion, thereby removing the negative feedback control on gastrin secretion by G cells [6]. Hypergastrinemia in MEN1/ZES results from ectopic secretion of gastrin from a gastrinoma found in the pancreas or duodenum. In MEN1/ZES, a finding of significance has been the loss of heterozygosity at chromosome 11q13 exhibited in all type II gastric carcinoids. This loss of heterozygosity can also be seen infrequently with type I and III gastric carcinoids. Interestingly, gastric carcinoid is 70 times as common in MEN1/ZES than in sporadic ZES, which reflects an underlying genetic contributor [8]. Hypergastrinemia alone is likely not the sole cause of ECL cell transformation, since gastrin decreasing measures, such as vagotomy and chronic proton-pump inhibition, do not lead to increased risk of gastric carcinoid development. Other potential cofactors involve environmental changes, growth factors, bacterial infections, and effects on underlying mesenchyme [3]. Reg, a growth factor secreted by both ECL and chief cells, has been under study, as it is known to be increased in gastric carcinoids. This growth factor has a role in the feedback mechanism that restrains the stimulating effects of gastrin and, therefore, mutations in Reg would lead to unrestrained gastrin effects [12].

Although discrete models of tumor progression originating with ECL cells have been proposed in both type I and II gastric carcinoids, there are still many unanswered questions. The Mastomys rodent is a prototype species of gastrointestinal carcinoid in that these rodents will spontaneously develop gastric carcinoids in the setting of pharmacologic acid suppression and consequent hypergastrinemia [10]. In humans, long-term pharmacologic acid suppression has not yet shown a similar effect [11].

Little is known regarding the pathogenesis of type III gastric carcinoid, although overexpression or a mutation in p53, a tumor suppression gene, is present in a large majority of tumors [13].

6.5 Diagnosis

Gastric carcinoids are usually diagnosed by upper gastrointestinal endoscopy and direct visualization of the stomach. Whether or not to offer surveillance endoscopy to patients with CAG is controversial, but it is recommended for MEN1 patients every 2–3 years [5]. Lesions generally appear as small, multiple, rounded submucosal erythematous nodules that can be yellowish in color (see Fig. 6.2). Larger lesions will be solitary and sometimes ulcerated. Once suspected, biopsies of both the lesion and the surrounding gastric mucosa should be performed. Gastric mapping of the surrounding mucosa will determine whether or not there is CAG, which will help to differentiate type I gastric carcinoid from the other two types. The biopsies should be stained for chromogranin A and synaptophysin, which are markers for ECL cells. Immunohistochemical analysis for Ki-67 index and mitotic count is mandatory to determine histologic grade. A useful serologic marker for diagnosis is chromogranin A. Chromogranin A has a sensitivity of >90 % and correlates well with tumor burden, especially when metastasized to the liver. Frequently, chromogranin A is used as a surveillance marker to monitor progression of disease. However, chromogranin A is not specific to carcinoid and can be found in ECL cell hyperplasia and hypergastrinemia alone. In patients presenting with symptoms of carcinoid syndrome, a 24-h urine 5-hydroxylindoleacetic acid (5-HIAA) is the test of choice [3, 12]. Atypical carcinoid syndrome arises due

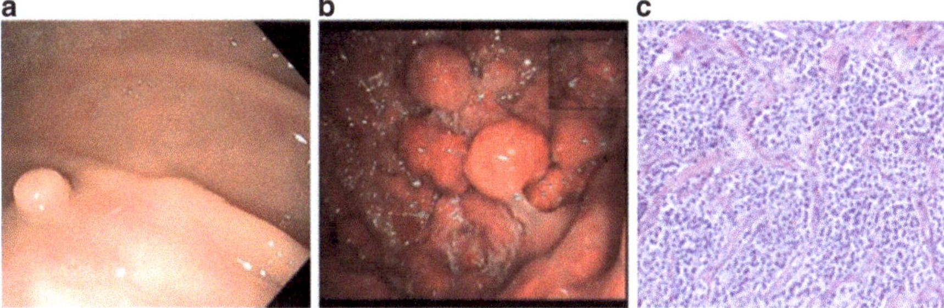

Fig. 6.2 Endoscopic and histologic appearance of gastric carcinoid. (**a**) Less than 1 cm type III gastric carcinoid tumor in the gastric fundus seen on incidental endoscopy. (**b**) Multiple type II gastric carcinoids in a patient with MEN1/ZES. (**c**) Type II gastric carcinoid with nested insular pattern, fine trabeculae, and monotonous nuclei, which are hallmark of carcinoids

to deficiency of the enzyme dopa-decarboxylase, which is responsible for the conversion of 5-hydroxytryptophan to 5-hydroxytryptamine (serotonin). Therefore, in atypical carcinoid syndrome, the precursor, 5-hydroxytryptophan, is elevated instead [9].

Further diagnostic testing is imperative to determine the type of gastric carcinoid. A serum gastrin level (off anti-acid therapy) should be the first step in differentiating between gastrin-dependent and gastrin-independent tumor. If gastrin is elevated and there is no prior diagnosis of atrophic gastritis, a complete blood count and vitamin B12 level are helpful, with further testing for antibodies against parietal cells and intrinsic factor if pernicious anemia is suspected. Gastric mapping by mucosal biopsy should be done to determine if there is atrophic gastritis and ECL cell hyperplasia, which would support type I gastric carcinoid. To evaluate for type II gastric carcinoid, serum gastrin and gastric pH levels are used for the diagnosis of MEN1/ZES. If serum gastrin is greater than 1,000 and gastric pH is less than 2, the diagnosis of ZES is definite. If testing is indeterminate with a gastrin between 100 and 1,000 and pH less than 2, a secretin test should be ordered and completed off pharmacologic acid suppression for at least 5–8 days. For patients newly diagnosed with MEN1/ZES, genetic testing for a mutation in the *MENIN* gene is available, and further evaluation for parathyroid, pancreatic, and pituitary tumors is warranted. When serum gastrin levels are normal and no atrophy is noted on gastric biopsies, the tumor under evaluation is likely to be type III or sporadic in origin. Histological analysis may reveal a Ki-67 level greater than 2 %, which can differentiate type III from type I and II gastric carcinoids. A small proportion of patients with gastrinomas have normal fasting serum gastrin concentrations and a secretin test can be performed to rule out MEN1/ZES before type III GC is confirmed [2, 5, 10].

Adjunctive testing to upper endoscopy may be recommended in the appropriate setting. Endoscopic ultrasound (EUS) is the best technique to evaluate tumor size, infiltration, and regional lymph node enlargement and can be considered in tumors greater than 1 cm. If there is evidence of invasion or concern for regional or distant metastasis in type I and II gastric carcinoids, computed tomography (CT) should be obtained to evaluate for liver metastasis. An abdominal and thoracic CT is required for type III gastric carcinoid. For better evaluation of diffuse or smaller lesions undetectable with imaging, a functional study called somatostatin receptor scintigraphy (SRS), also known as octreoscan, is useful in localizing areas of disease. Approximately 85 % of gastric carcinoids express somatostatin receptors. With SRS, octreotide radiolabeled with indium-111 is injected into the bloodstream and nuclear images are taken. SRS should be performed in all patients with type III and sparingly in invasive type I and II gastric carcinoids [3–5, 9, 10]. SRS has better sensitivity and specificity as compared to CT, but several limitations should be kept in mind. It does not detect 10–15 % of tumors that do not express somatostatin receptors, the detection size limit is 0.5 cm, and there is relatively poor anatomic localization [12].

6.6 Treatment

A spectrum of modalities for treatment of gastric carcinoids exists from endoscopic removal to complete gastrectomy (see Fig. 6.3). Management of gastric carcinoid differs considerably with the type, grade, and stage of tumor.

6.6.1 *Type I and II*

The principle of treatment for type I gastric carcinoid is to minimize risk given the lack of increased mortality with disease. For lesions limited to the submucosa, smaller than 1 cm, and fewer than five in total, endoscopic mucosal resection (EMR) is sufficient. Some clinicians may opt for conservative treatment with annual endoscopic surveillance given the low risk for local or distant metastasis, particularly in elderly patients. Treatment of lesions between 1 and 2 cm and greater than five in number is controversial with no controlled studies thus far comparing different methods. EMR is an acceptable technique with close surveillance endoscopy every 6 months initially, then annually after 3 years. If recurrence is found, either repeat EMR can be attempted or the patient can be referred for surgical evaluation for

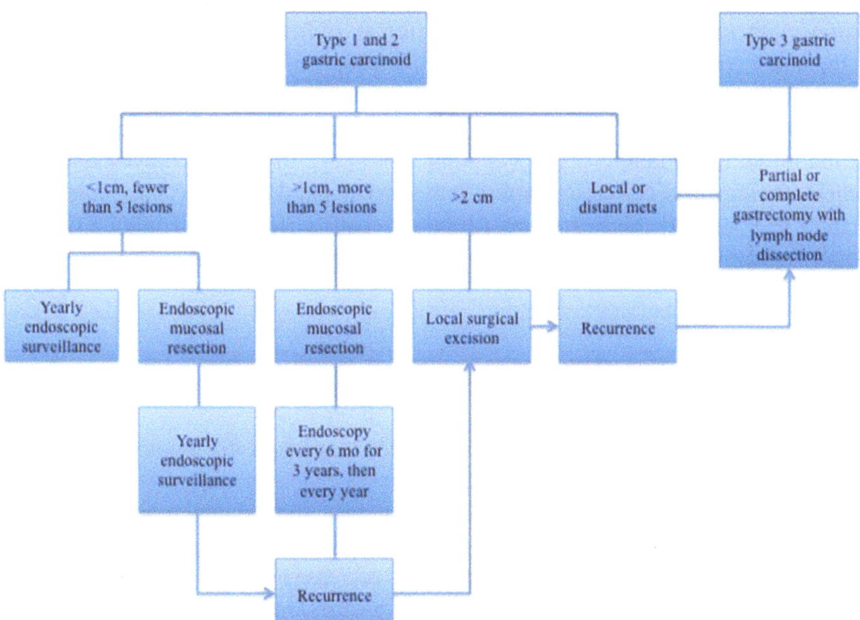

Fig. 6.3 Algorithm of treatment of gastric carcinoid by type

excision or even gastrectomy. Local surgical resection is recommended in patients with lesions greater than 2 cm and should be strongly considered if the tumor is of higher grade or demonstrates invasion into the muscularis layer or blood vessels. Fundic resection with removal of all ECL cells and carcinoid tumors can be considered in young patients and those with large or multicentric tumors, as it would obviate the need for lifetime surveillance endoscopy. There has also been some success with antrectomy to eliminate the trophic stimulus of gastrin and therefore generate regression of tumors. However, this technique has not been reliable due to the concern for gastrin autonomous lesions. 70–85 % of patients have tumor regression at 3- and 5-year follow-up while remaining patients have tumor recurrence or persistence. Management of type II gastric carcinoids is similar to type I although its greater potential for regional and distant spread should be noted. Removal of the gastrin stimulus can also be achieved in type II gastric carcinoids with surgical gastrinoma excision. Unfortunately, gastrinomas are typically multiple and many patients have lymph node metastasis at the time of surgery [4, 5, 12].

6.6.2 *Type III*

Unlike type I and II gastric carcinoids, management of type III gastric carcinoid is straightforward. Aggressive surgical management with complete or partial gastrectomy with regional lymph node dissection is indicated in almost all tumors. One study correlated tumor size and depth with rate of lymph node metastasis and concluded that local or endoscopic resection for type III gastric carcinoid may be appropriate for intraepithelial tumors less than 2 cm and perhaps tumors less than 1 cm invading the lamina propria or submucosa [14]. In poor operative candidates, chemotherapy may increase progress-free survival but does not produce substantial tumor response [9]. Also, in select patients, hepatic chemoembolization, cryoablation, or radiofrequency ablation can be performed on liver lesions.

6.6.3 *Alternative Options*

Nonsurgical management of gastric carcinoid is less frequently employed, but is an option in type I and II gastric carcinoids. Therapy with long-acting octreotide, a somatostatin analog, induces a rapid fall in serum gastrin and chromogranin A due to an inhibitory effect on ECL cell function. Intramuscular treatments are given on a monthly basis. During treatment, gastrin levels decrease by 50 %; however, long-term follow-up has shown a return to pretreatment gastrin levels along with no mortality benefit. There is also a concern for a rebound effect with disease progression after discontinuation, prompting the suggestion that octreotide treatment should not be stopped if initiated. Furthermore, the high cost of therapy precludes use in many patients and is not practical from a cost-effectiveness standpoint [15]. Other experimental treatments on the horizon include a specific gastrin receptor (CCK2) antagonist, a vaccine against gastrin, and antibodies against pro-gastrin-releasing peptide [3, 9]. One current ongoing clinical trial in patients with MEN1/ZES is studying YF476, a gastrin antagonist, which may block the effects of gastrinomas and reduce the need for surgical management of type II gastric carcinoids [16]. These novel agents, although promising, need further study to substantiate clinical utility.

References

1. Wardlaw R, Smith JW. Gastric carcinoid tumors. Oschsner J. 2008;8:191–6.
2. Modlin IM, Lye KD, Kidd M. A 50-year analysis of 562 gastric carcinoids: small tumor or larger problem? Am J Gastroenterol. 2004;99(1):23–32.
3. Nikou GC, Angelopoulos TP. Current concepts on gastric carcinoid tumors. Gastroenterol Res Pract. 2012;2012:287825.
4. Modlin IM, Kidd M, Latich I, Zikusoka MN, Shapiro MD. Current status of gastrointestinal carcinoids. Gastroenterology. 2005;128:1717–51.
5. Scherubl H, Cadlot G, Jensen RT, Rosch T, Stolzel U, Kloppel G. Neuroendocrine tumors of the stomach (gastric carcinoids) are on the rise: small tumors, small problems? Endoscopy. 2010;42(8):664–71.
6. Hagarty S, Huttner I, Shibata H, Katz S. Gastric carcinoid tumours and pernicious anemia: case report and review of the literature. Can J Gastroenterol. 2000;14(3):241–5.
7. Vannella L, Lahner E, Annibale B. Risk for gastric neoplasias in patients with chronic atrophic gastritis: a critical appraisal. World J Gastroenterol. 2012;18(12):1279–85.
8. Berna MJ, Annibale B, Marignani M, Luong TV, Corleto V, Pace A, et al. A prospective study of gastric carcinoids and enterochrommafin-like cell changes in multiple endocrine neoplasia type 1 and Zollinger-Ellison syndrome: identification of risk factors. J Clin Endocrinol Metab. 2008;93(5):1582–91.
9. Kidd M, Gustafsson BI. Management of gastric carcinoids (neuroendocrine neoplasms). Curr Gastroenterol Rep. 2012;14:467–72.
10. Burkitt MD, Prichard DM. Review article: pathogenesis and management of gastric carcinoid tumours. Aliment Pharmacol Ther. 2006;24(9):1305–20.
11. Thomson AB, Sauve MD, Kassam N, Kamitakahara H. Safety of the long-term use of proton pump inhibitors. World J Gastroenterol. 2010;16(19):2323–30.
12. Zhang L, Ozao J, Warner R, Divino C. Review of the pathogenesis, diagnosis, and management of type I gastric carcinoid tumor. World J Surg. 2011;35:1879–86.
13. Delle Fave G, Capurso G, Milione M, Panzuto F. Endocrine tumours of the stomach. Best Pract Res Clin Gastroenterol. 2005;19(5):659–73.
14. Saund MS, Al Natour RH, Sharma AM, Huang Q, Boosalis VA, Gold JS. Tumor size and depth predict rate of lymph node metastasis and utilization of lymph node sampling in surgically managed gastric carcinoids. Ann Surg Oncol. 2011;18:2826–32.
15. Jianu CS, Fossmark R, Syversen U, Hauso O, Fykse V, Waldum HI. Five-year follow-up of patients treated for 1 year with octreotide long-acting release for enterochromaffin-like cell carcinoids. Scand J Gastroenterol. 2011;46(4):456–63.
16. NIH Clinical Research Studies [internet]. A pilot trial of YF476, a gastrin antagonist, in patients with type II gastric carcinoids associated with Zollinger-Ellison syndrome [updated 2013 May 29; cited 2013 May 29]. http://clinicalstudies.info.nih.gov/cgi/wais/bold032001.pl?A_11-DK-0114.html@carcinoid
17. Oates JA, Sjoerdsma A. A unique syndrome associated with secretion of 5-hydroxytryptophan by metastatic gastric carcinoids. Am J Med. 1962;32(3):333–42.

Chapter 7
Endoscopic Approaches for Diagnosis of Pancreatic Neuroendocrine Tumors

Tarun Rustagi and James J. Farrell

7.1 Introduction

Pancreatic neuroendocrine tumors (PNETs) are rare pancreatic neoplasms comprising only 1–2 % of all pancreatic tumors with an annual incidence of 1–5 cases per million in the United States [1–6]. They may occur sporadically or in association with a genetic syndrome, such as multiple endocrine neoplasia type 1 (MEN1), von Hippel–Lindau (VHL) syndrome, neurofibromatosis type 1, or tuberous sclerosis [4, 7–9]. PNETs typically have a more indolent course with a much better overall prognosis and long-term survival compared to exocrine pancreatic cancers [10, 11].

PNETs are usually well-differentiated tumors divided into two groups: those associated with a functional syndrome due to ectopic secretion of a biologically active substance (called "functional" PNETs [F-PNETs]) and those that are not associated with a functional syndrome (generally called "nonfunctional" PNETs [NF-PNETs]) [1–4, 12–14]. As a result of their biochemical activity, F-PNETs are usually detected at small sizes. In contrast, NF-PNETs may be found incidentally or present with symptoms related to a mass effect of the tumor or metastases, and as such NF-PNETs are usually discovered at larger sizes compared with F-PNETs [14]. With the widespread use of axial imaging, an increasing number of asymptomatic PNETs are being detected incidentally [2, 15].

T. Rustagi, M.D. • J.J. Farrell, M.D. (✉)
Yale Center for Pancreatic Disease, Yale University School of Medicine, LMP 1080, 15 York Street, New Haven, CT 06510-3221, USA

Section of Digestive Diseases, Yale University School of Medicine, LMP 1080, 15 York Street, New Haven, CT 06510-3221, USA
e-mail: tarun.rustagi@yale.edu; james.j.farrell@yale.edu

J.R. Pisegna (ed.), *Management of Pancreatic Neuroendocrine Tumors*,
DOI 10.1007/978-1-4939-1798-3_7

7.2 Diagnostic Endoscopic Ultrasound

The close proximity of the pancreas to the gastric and duodenal wall particularly lends itself to detailed examination via EUS. The head of the pancreas and the uncinate process can be visualized transduodenally, whereas the neck, body, and tail are seen through the stomach wall. The pancreatic parenchyma, ducts, and vasculature can be well visualized. Additionally, adjacent celiac, peripancreatic, para-aortic, and periportal lymphadenopathy can also be seen and evaluated. Unlike other imaging studies such as CT, MRI, and SRS, EUS is well suited to the identification of small pancreatic lesions, as small as 2–5 mm [16, 17].

The seminal article by Rosch et al. in 1992 was the first to describe the important role of EUS in the detection of PNETs [16]. In this study, EUS demonstrated a sensitivity of 82 % and a specificity of 92 % in the detection of islet cell tumors in 50 patients with previously undetected tumors by radiological imaging [16]. Since then, EUS has been increasingly used and has become an integral part of the diagnosis of PNETs because of its high sensitivity for detecting, localizing, and diagnosing pancreatic PNETs [18, 19]. EUS is particularly useful in the detection of smaller insulinomas, where other modalities such as SRS have low sensitivity. The average size of insulinomas at initial diagnosis is 6–10 mm, with 75 % of lesions smaller than 15 mm, which is well within the detection capability of EUS [17, 20]. PNETs may be multifocal in up to 9 % of cases, and smaller, synchronous lesions may not be detected by CT and seen only on EUS [21].

Most commonly, PNETs appear as round, well-demarcated, homogeneous, hypoechoic lesions within the pancreas. However, some PNETs may be isoechoic, and, on rare occasions, hyperechoic with irregular margins. Isoechoic PNETs may be difficult to distinguish from normal pancreatic parenchyma. Malignant PNETs are usually larger, with irregular margins, compared to the benign PNETs. The presence of isoechogenicity or hyperechogenicity, vascular invasion, and pancreatic duct obstruction has been shown to be predictive of malignant PNETs [22, 23]. Additionally, EUS–FNA may detect and confirm the presence of malignant lymph nodes and liver metastases previously unseen on cross-sectional imaging [24].

While the majority of PNETs are solid, 8–21 % of PNETs present as thin-walled cysts with variable degrees of focal or concentric wall thickening [25–30]. Cystic PNETs may present a diagnostic challenge to the endosonographer as they may be difficult to distinguish from much more common cystic lesions such as pseudocysts or mucinous cystic neoplasms [26, 29, 31, 32]. Cystic PNETs may be unilocular, septated, microcystic, or mixed solid-cystic in appearance with a normal surrounding pancreatic parenchyma and a normal main pancreatic duct [25–27]. Cystic PNETs are more often asymptomatic, more likely to be associated with genetic (MEN-1, VHL) syndromes, and twice as large (median cyst size was 35 mm [range 8–80 mm] in one study), compared to their solid counterparts [18, 25, 29, 33].

Majority of cystic PNETs (81 %) are nonfunctional [26], and diagnosis with radiological or EUS imaging alone is likely to be inaccurate or nondiagnostic [32],

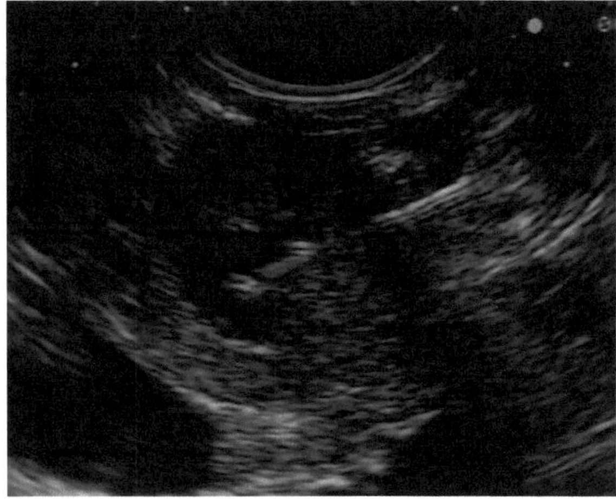

Fig. 7.1 Endoscopic ultrasound fine-needle aspiration (EUS-FNA) of a 2-cm pancreatic head cystic neuroendocrine tumor

given the lack of distinguishing features of these cystic lesions. Therefore, cytologic and immunohistochemical evaluation of EUS–FNA specimens is essential for diagnosing cystic PNETs and appears to have similar sensitivity as the EUS–FNA of solid PNETs [34]. In one study, EUS–FNA demonstrated immunocytological features of PNETs in all 13 cystic PNET patients, compared to CT imaging that demonstrated typical features of PNETs (peripheral hypervascularity) in only three of the 13 patients [35]. This was revisited by a recent retrospective, multicenter series of 27 patients in which cystic PNETs were suspected in only 2 (7.4 %) patients based on presenting symptoms prior to endosonography, suggesting that a high degree of suspicion is required among endosonographers to recognize these lesions [29]. EUS–FNA cytology confirmed neuroendocrine tumor in 17 of 24 (71 %) patients. Targeting the wall during FNA was found to have a higher diagnostic yield of EUS–FNA cytology (88.9 % vs. 66.7 % without wall targeting) and, therefore, should be performed in all possible cases (Fig. 7.1) [29]. Cyst fluid is typically nonviscous with very low carcinoembryonic antigen levels [29].

7.3 Diagnostic Accuracy of Endoscopic Ultrasound

Studies evaluating the diagnostic accuracy of EUS predominantly focus on detection of F-PNETs that are frequently detected biochemically. Given that more than 90 % of insulinomas are located in the pancreas and that up to 90 % of insulinomas are less than 2 cm, EUS is well suited for their detection. Numerous studies on accuracy of EUS, particularly in the detection of insulinomas, have been published with detection rates ranging from 79 to 94 % [36–38]. A study on 52 patients undergoing EUS for detection of a suspected insulinoma (based on clinical and laboratory findings) reported a sensitivity of 89.5 % and accuracy of 83.7 % based on surgical findings [39]. Similar to previous data, this study found EUS to be more sensitive for detecting tumors in the head and body compared to the tail (92.6, 78.9, and 40.0 %, for pancreatic head, body, and tail, respectively) [39].

A recent meta-analysis of 13 studies ($n=456$) showed a high-pooled sensitivity and specificity of EUS in detecting PNETs, 87.2 % (95% CI, 82.2–91.2) and 98.0 % (95% CI, 94.3–99.6), respectively [40]. Overall, EUS had a high positive likelihood ratio of 11.1 (95% CI, 5.34–22.8) and a low negative likelihood ratio of 0.17 (95% CI, 0.13–0.24), making it an excellent diagnostic test. Summary receiver operating characteristic (SROC) curves showed an area under the curve of 0.94 [40]. EUS as a diagnostic test has a very high diagnostic odds ratio (DOR), the odds of having anatomic PNETs in positive as compared to negative EUS studies, to detect PNETs (about 95 times). If EUS localizes the lesion to the pancreas, the odds of having the correct histological neuroendocrine tumor in the pancreas is 95 times [40].

Authors also performed a subgroup analysis to evaluate EUS performance in detecting an insulinoma or a gastrinoma in the pancreas. In line with the prior literature, pancreatic gastrinomas were found to have detection rates similar to that of insulinomas (pooled sensitivity and specificity of 84.5 and 95.3 % compared to 87.5 and 97.4 %, for pancreatic gastrinoma and insulinoma, respectively) [40, 41]. However, EUS detection rates have been reported to be disappointingly low (11–50 %) for gastrinomas located outside the pancreas (extrapancreatic), which comprise 50 % of all gastrinomas, likely due to their smaller size at presentation [42, 43]. A distinct advantage of EUS in these patients, however, is in detection of adjacent metastatic lymph nodes within the "gastrinoma triangle," which may alter treatment strategies [42]. In addition, as extrapancreatic gastrinomas are located primarily in the duodenum, a careful optical inspection of duodenal wall combined with excessive biopsy of any suspected lesion should be performed during esophagogastroduodenoscopy (EGD) to increase the rate of detection [42].

Detection of PNETs by EUS has potential pitfalls, including very small lesions, multiple lesions, isoechoic appearance, and pedunculated lesions at the pancreatic tail [44]. Female gender, low body mass index, and young age have been reported as risk factors for a negative EUS, likely due to weak contrast of the tumor to healthy pancreatic tissue, which in slim young women may be more hypoechoic than usual due to low fat content [45]. In addition, because PNETs may be multifocal, it is important to examine the entire pancreas to exclude a synchronous lesion [17, 21].

7.4 EUS-Guided Tissue Acquisition of PNETs

There are multiple techniques used to obtain tissue confirmation of PNETs. The most commonly used is EUS-guided fine-needle aspiration (EUS–FNA).

7.4.1 EUS-Guided Fine-Needle Aspiration

EUS-guided FNA is an excellent diagnostic tool to detect the correct etiology for solid and cystic pancreatic lesions. Similar to other pancreatic lesions, PNETs may be further evaluated by sampling these tumors by FNA performed during the EUS examination to optimize patient management (Fig. 7.2). Using a 22- or 25-gauge needle, endosonographers may obtain an aspirate that can be evaluated for cytological features and immunohistochemistry. Ideally, onsite cytopathology evaluation is performed during the procedure to improve the yield and cost-effectiveness as it significantly reduces the rate of unsatisfactory cytology specimens from 20 to 9 % [46, 47]. If a cytopathologist is unavailable, 5–7 needle passes for a pancreatic tumor, 2–3 for liver metastases, and 2–5 for lymph nodes are recommended to ensure adequate FNA samples for analysis [48, 49]. The diagnosis is generally confirmed with immunohistochemical studies from the cell block. Most commonly performed immunostains include chromogranin and synaptophysin; other stains may include neuron-specific enolase (NSE), CD56, and CDX (Fig. 7.3) [2, 50, 51].

EUS–FNA is the diagnostic modality of choice for the diagnosis of PNETs, owing to its high sensitivity and specificity [34]. Studies have reported sensitivities of 61–84 % and overall accuracy of up to 92.5 % of EUS–FNA in establishing the diagnosis of PNETs [34, 52, 53]. Additionally, FNA may detect and confirm the presence of malignant lymph nodes and liver metastases previously unseen on CT imaging [24, 53].

Alternative methods for obtaining a tissue via EUS have been evaluated to overcome the limitations of FNA. The core needle or Tru-Cut needle biopsy uses a 19-, 22-, or 25-gauge needle to obtain core biopsies with the benefit of a more substantive specimen to provide cellular architecture for pathologic analysis (Fig. 7.4).

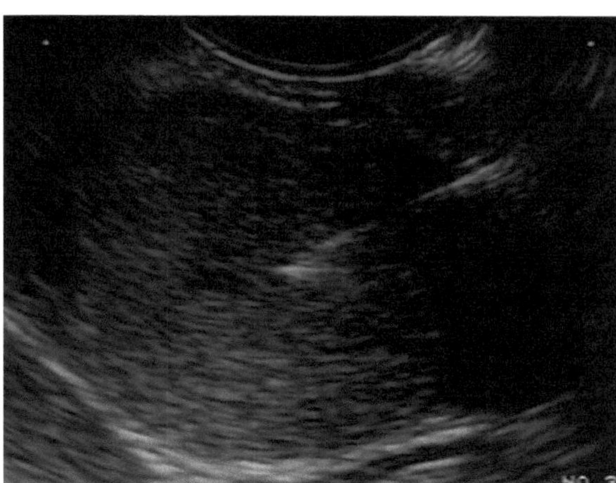

Fig. 7.2 Endoscopic ultrasound fine-needle aspiration (EUS-FNA) of a 3-cm pancreatic tail neuroendocrine tumor

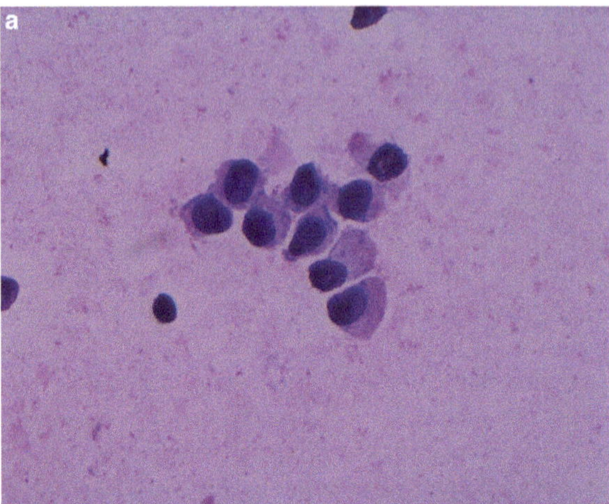

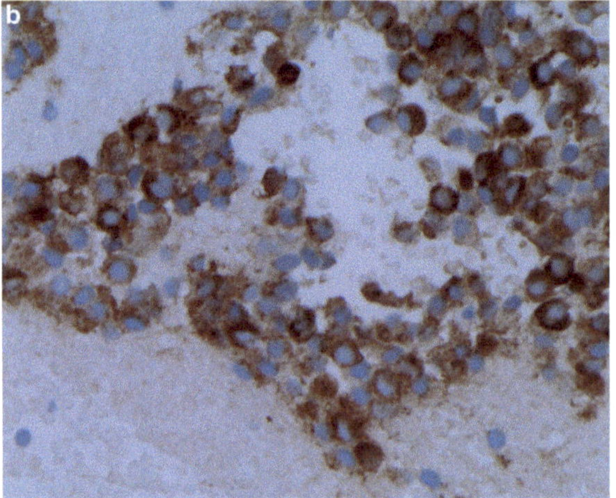

Fig. 7.3 Endoscopic ultrasound fine-needle aspiration cytology. (**a**) Typical plasmacytoid appearance of a pancreatic NET with eccentrically located nuclei and finely granular cytoplasm (Diff-Quik stain, 600×). (**b**) Immunocytochemistry of a pancreatic NET staining positive (*brown*) for chromogranin (400×)

Combining EUS–FNA and Tru-Cut needle biopsy may increase the overall sensitivity of pancreatic mass sampling [54]; however, studies have not consistently demonstrated superior diagnostic yield, and this has not been adequately studied for PNETs. In addition, the use of the core needle has been limited by the technical difficulties of using this device, particularly with the duodenal approach [55]. Therefore, lesions in the pancreatic head and uncinate process are difficult to access, and, again, there is inadequate data with PNETs.

For evaluation of cystic PNETs, EUS-guided brushing may provide superior diagnostic yield to FNA [56, 57]; however, increased risk of bleeding and difficulty in performing the technique from the duodenum may preclude this from more widespread use [56, 57].

In addition to facilitating diagnosis of PNETs, EUS-guided tissue acquisition may allow prognostication about tumor behavior. Typical markers of malignancy may be seen including presence or absence of necrosis and mitotic index. Nodit and

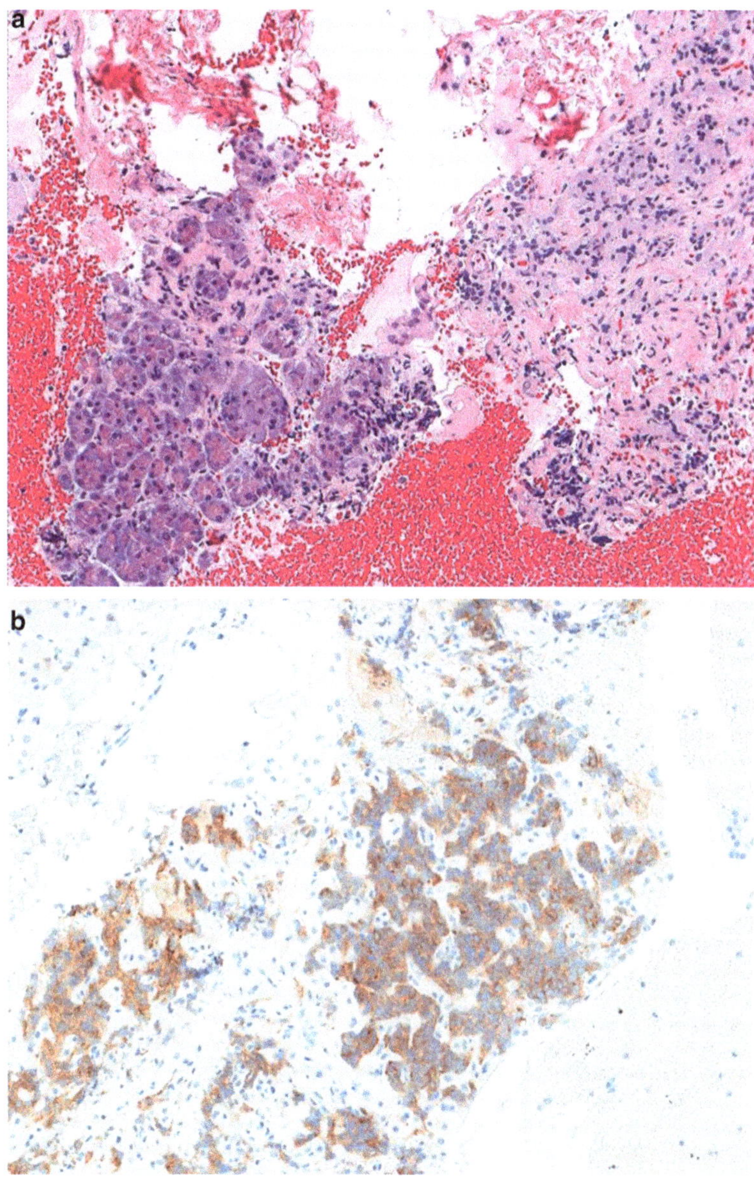

Fig. 7.4 Endoscopic ultrasound-guided fine-needle core biopsy: (**a**) Histologic core biopsy showing uniform cells consistent with a pancreatic endocrine neoplasm (H&E stain). (**b**) Immunohistochemistry stain with synaptophysin (*brown*) supporting the diagnosis of pancreatic endocrine neoplasm

colleagues reported a significant difference in the profiles of benign and malignant PNETs as well as of progressive and stable PNETs based on the results of microsatellite loss analysis of cellular aspirates obtained from EUS–FNA [58]. Another study demonstrated the feasibility of measuring Ki-67 expression (proliferative index), a powerful marker of malignant behavior, on cytological specimens obtained by EUS–FNA [59]. This information is particularly important as it may aid in the grading of PNETs and provide prognostic information which might be of great help for further therapeutic decisions.

7.5 EUS for Screening and Surveillance

7.5.1 *MEN Type 1 Patients*

MEN-1 patients have a high incidence of PNETs, ranging from 36 to 81 % [2]. NF-PNETs, which may account for 20–50 % of PNETs in these patients, are typically found at late stages and represent the main source of morbidity and mortality. Given the high incidence of PNETs, and potential malignant complications, EUS surveillance programs have been proposed to detect PNETs at early stages in MEN-1 patients (Fig. 7.5). A surveillance study of 51 asymptomatic MEN-1 patients reported the incidence of pancreatic tumors to be 54.9 %. The median number of PNETs per patient was 3, with a median size of 6 mm. 37.5 % of patients who underwent repeat EUS developed additional or enlarging tumors or both, over a mean of 50 months [60]. The usefulness of a similar EUS surveillance program for detecting small asymptomatic PNETs in MEN-1 patients was further evaluated in a study by Kann et al., which followed 20 patients with a total of 82 tumors (all <15 mm) over a period of 20 months [61]. The increase in the largest tumor diameter was 1.3 % per month, with an annual tumor incidence rate of 0.62 tumors per patient. No patients developed evidence of metastatic disease. One patient developed rapidly progressive tumor burden. Less than 10 % of all tumors were detected by CT, MRI, or SRS. These studies indicate that EUS is a useful tool for detecting and monitoring small pancreatic tumors in MEN-1 patients; however, the long-term benefit in outcomes such as survival remains to be seen.

7.5.2 *Nonoperative Management of Small NF-PNETs*

As significant proportion of non-MEN-1 patients with small NF-PNETs may exhibit minimal or no growth over many years, controversy exists regarding the optimal management of such incidentally discovered tumors. A recent study of 77 NF-PNET patients with a median tumor size of 1.0 cm (range, 0.3–3.2) reported no change in median tumor size and no disease progression or disease-specific mortality over a mean follow-up of 45 months [62]. EUS can be helpful in serial follow-up of these patients to detect growth or suspicious features necessitating surgical resection.

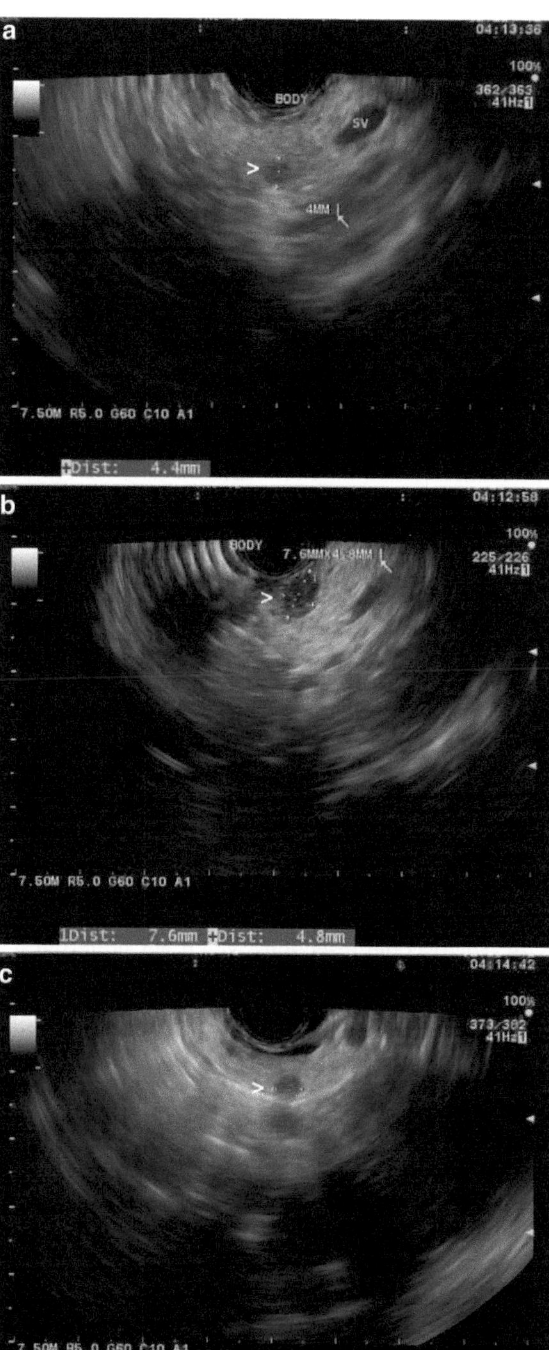

Fig. 7.5 A 40-year-old male with MEN-1 syndrome and normal imaging of pancreas with MRI and CT. (**a**)–(**c**) Endoscopic ultrasound of pancreas shows three distinct isolated sub-centimeter pancreatic masses consistent with multifocal pancreatic endocrine neoplasm

7.6 Preoperative EUS

EUS is useful in the preoperative assessment of PNETs by providing information that significantly influences the decision for surgical intervention or changes the extent of the planned surgery. In one study, EUS altered the decision for possible surgical management in five of 14 patients (36 %), either by identifying a PNET or by finding multiple and multifocal PNETs that were not visualized on CT scan [63]. Another study evaluating preoperative assessment of the pancreas in 52 MEN-1 patients found preoperative CT to have 81 % sensitivity and scintigraphy to have 84 % sensitivity compared to preoperative EUS which was found to have 100 % sensitivity with close correlation (*rs* = 0.93) between the largest lesion seen on EUS and pathology [64].

Preoperative EUS is not only the most sensitive modality for diagnosis of insulinoma but is helpful in assessing the candidacy for enucleation, by imaging the proximity of the mass to the main pancreatic duct (Fig. 7.6) [65, 66]. Accurate preoperative localization of insulinomas by EUS may favor enucleation over blind distal pancreatectomy, eliminating the need for more extensive surgical resection and avoiding the need for surgical re-exploration [65]. In addition, EUS can also evaluate the presence of multiple insulinomas and metastases to the liver or lymph nodes, which will preclude enucleation.

7.7 Improving Intraoperative Localization

Small PNETs may be difficult to localize in the operating room. Intraoperative palpation combined with intraoperative ultrasound is over 95 % sensitive; however, it prolongs operative time, can rarely cause splenic vessel rupture, and is not practical with laparoscopic resections which are preferred for small lesions [67]. This has prompted efforts for better preoperative localization via EUS interventions. The safety and efficacy of EUS-guided fine-needle injection (FNI) of PNETs for endoscopic

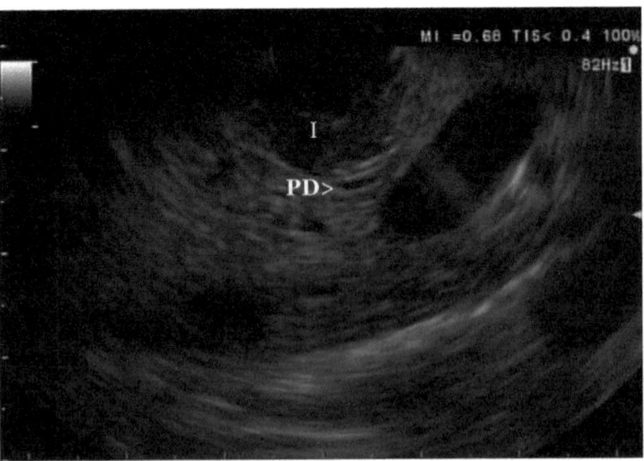

Fig. 7.6 Endoscopic ultrasound demonstrating close proximity between a clinically and pathologically confirmed insulinoma (I) and a normal caliber main pancreatic duct (PD)

tattooing have been described in small case series [68, 69]. The agents such as diluted India ink, indocyanine green, and GI Spot are typically injected into the pancreas few hours prior to surgery [68–70].

Recently, EUS-guided fiducial placement has also been described to aid precise intraoperative localization of small PNETs. Law and colleagues reported two successful cases where VISICOIL fiducials (Core Oncology, Santa Barbara, CA, USA) were placed either within or adjacent to the small (7 and 9 mm) tumors using a 22-gauge Cook EchoTip needle prior to parenchyma-sparing pancreatic surgery [71].

7.8 New Technology

Recently, there has been a development of adjunctive techniques with EUS to further increase potential detection of small lesions. Contrast-enhanced harmonic EUS (CEH–EUS) is one such technique with most common clinical application including the differential diagnosis of focal pancreatic masses, with adenocarcinoma having a distinct hypovascular (hypo-enhanced) appearance compared with neuroendocrine tumors, which are hypervascular (with strong arterial hyper-enhancement) [72–74]. Recent studies have reported a higher sensitivity of EUS in combination with CEH–EUS for the diagnosis of PNETs compared with multidetector CT [19, 74]. In one recent Japanese study, CEH–EUS-depicted hypervascular enhancement diagnosed neuroendocrine tumors with a sensitivity and specificity of 78.9 % (95 % CI, 61.4–89.7) and 98.7 % (95 % CI, 96.7–98.8), respectively [74]. When CEH–EUS was combined with EUS–FNA, the sensitivity of EUS–FNA increased from 92.2 to 100 % [74].

Another technique is EUS elastography combined with the strain ratio of tissue elasticity for diagnosis of solid pancreatic masses. One study reported different scores, in which score 4 represented a hypoechoic region in the center, with a green appearance within a small area surrounded by blue, or harder tissue, corresponding to neuroendocrine tumors [75]. However, in this study, the association between score 4 and PNET was only 33.3 % [75]. In another study, all 6 neuroendocrine tumors consistently showed a homogeneous blue elastographic pattern [76]. Endocrine tumors as a group presented the lowest elasticity value and highest strain ratio [76]. EUS elastography was reported to be helpful for differentiating pancreatic cancer from neuroendocrine tumors with a sensitivity of 100 % and specificity close to 88 % [76].

References

1. Oberg K, Eriksson B. Endocrine tumours of the pancreas. Best Pract Res Clin Gastroenterol. 2005;19:753–81.
2. Rustagi T, Rai M, Bauer F. Non-functional pancreatic neuroendocrine tumor as an incidentaloma—a case report and review of literature. J Gastrointest Cancer. 2013;44:336–42.

3. Kloppel G, Anlauf M. Epidemiology, tumour biology and histopathological classification of neuroendocrine tumours of the gastrointestinal tract. Best Pract Res Clin Gastroenterol. 2005;19:507–17.
4. Metz DC, Jensen RT. Gastrointestinal neuroendocrine tumors: pancreatic endocrine tumors. Gastroenterology. 2008;135:1469–92.
5. Halfdanarson TR, Rabe KG, Rubin J, Petersen GM. Pancreatic neuroendocrine tumors (PNETs): incidence, prognosis and recent trend toward improved survival. Ann Oncol. 2008;19:1727–33.
6. Fesinmeyer MD, Austin MA, Li CI, De Roos AJ, Bowen DJ. Differences in survival by histologic type of pancreatic cancer. Cancer Epidemiol Biomarkers Prev. 2005;14:1766–73.
7. Massironi S, Sciola V, Peracchi M, Ciafardini C, Spampatti MP, Conte D. Neuroendocrine tumors of the gastro-entero-pancreatic system. World J Gastroenterol. 2008;14:5377–84.
8. Jensen RT, Berna MJ, Bingham DB, Norton JA. Inherited pancreatic endocrine tumor syndromes: advances in molecular pathogenesis, diagnosis, management, and controversies. Cancer. 2008;113:1807–43.
9. Gibril F, Schumann M, Pace A, Jensen RT. Multiple endocrine neoplasia type 1 and Zollinger-Ellison syndrome: a prospective study of 107 cases and comparison with 1009 cases from the literature. Medicine (Baltimore). 2004;83:43–83.
10. Kang CM, Park SH, Kim KS, Choi JS, Lee WJ, Kim BR. Surgical experiences of functioning neuroendocrine neoplasm of the pancreas. Yonsei Med J. 2006;47:833–9.
11. Bilimoria KY, Talamonti MS, Tomlinson JS, et al. Prognostic score predicting survival after resection of pancreatic neuroendocrine tumors: analysis of 3851 patients. Ann Surg. 2008;247:490–500.
12. Ehehalt F, Saeger HD, Schmidt CM, Grutzmann R. Neuroendocrine tumors of the pancreas. Oncologist. 2009;14:456–67.
13. Falconi M, Plockinger U, Kwekkeboom DJ, et al. Well-differentiated pancreatic nonfunctioning tumors/carcinoma. Neuroendocrinology. 2006;84:196–211.
14. Bilimoria KY, Tomlinson JS, Merkow RP, et al. Clinicopathologic features and treatment trends of pancreatic neuroendocrine tumors: analysis of 9,821 patients. J Gastrointest Surg. 2007;11:1460–7. discussion 7-9.
15. Vagefi PA, Razo O, Deshpande V, et al. Evolving patterns in the detection and outcomes of pancreatic neuroendocrine neoplasms: the Massachusetts General Hospital experience from 1977 to 2005. Arch Surg. 2007;142:347–54.
16. Rosch T, Lightdale CJ, Botet JF, et al. Localization of pancreatic endocrine tumors by endoscopic ultrasonography. N Engl J Med. 1992;326:1721–6.
17. Kim MK. Endoscopic ultrasound in gastroenteropancreatic neuroendocrine tumors. Gut Liver. 2012;6:405–10.
18. Lee LS. Diagnosis of pancreatic neuroendocrine tumors and the role of endoscopic ultrasound. Gastroenterol Hepatol. 2010;6:520–2.
19. Ishikawa T, Itoh A, Kawashima H, et al. Usefulness of EUS combined with contrast-enhancement in the differential diagnosis of malignant versus benign and preoperative localization of pancreatic endocrine tumors. Gastrointest Endosc. 2010;71:951–9.
20. Akerstrom G, Hellman P. Surgery on neuroendocrine tumours. Best Pract Res Clin Endocrinol Metab. 2007;21:87–109.
21. Pais SAMK, Leblanc JK, et al. Clinical and endoscopic ultrasound morphology characteristics of pancreatic neuroendocrine tumors: a large, single center experience. Gastrointest Endosc. 2007;65:AB296.
22. Puli SR, Singh S, Hagedorn CH, Reddy J, Olyaee M. Diagnostic accuracy of EUS for vascular invasion in pancreatic and periampullary cancers: a meta-analysis and systematic review. Gastrointest Endosc. 2007;65:788–97.
23. Tox U, Hackenberg R, Stelzer A, et al. Endosonographic diagnosis of solid pancreatic tumors: a retrospective analysis from a tertiary referral center. Z Gastroenterol. 2007;45:307–12.
24. O'Neil JMA-HM, Leblanc J, et al. Endoscopic ultrasound morphology features and initial detection of metastatic liver lesions from primary pancreatic adenocarcinoma and pancreatic neuroendocrine carcinoma. Gastrointest Endosc. 2008;67:AB217–8.

25. Bordeianou L, Vagefi PA, Sahani D, et al. Cystic pancreatic endocrine neoplasms: a distinct tumor type? J Am Coll Surg. 2008;206:1154–8.
26. Kongkam P, Al-Haddad M, Attasaranya S, et al. EUS and clinical characteristics of cystic pancreatic neuroendocrine tumors. Endoscopy. 2008;40:602–5.
27. Goh BK, Ooi LL, Tan YM, et al. Clinico-pathological features of cystic pancreatic endocrine neoplasms and a comparison with their solid counterparts. Eur J Surg Oncol. 2006;32:553–6.
28. Buetow PC, Parrino TV, Buck JL, et al. Islet cell tumors of the pancreas: pathologic-imaging correlation among size, necrosis and cysts, calcification, malignant behavior, and functional status. AJR Am J Roentgenol. 1995;165:1175–9.
29. Ho HC, Eloubeidi MA, Siddiqui UD, et al. Endosonographic and cyst fluid characteristics of cystic pancreatic neuroendocrine tumours: a multicentre case series. Dig Liver Dis. 2013;45:750–3.
30. Jani N, Khalid A, Kaushik N, et al. EUS-guided FNA diagnosis of pancreatic endocrine tumors: new trends identified. Gastrointest Endosc. 2008;67:44–50.
31. Ahrendt SA, Komorowski RA, Demeure MJ, Wilson SD, Pitt HA. Cystic pancreatic neuroendocrine tumors: is preoperative diagnosis possible? J Gastrointest Surg. 2002;6:66–74.
32. Deshpande V, Lauwers GY. Cystic pancreatic endocrine tumor: a variant commonly confused with cystic adenocarcinoma. Cancer. 2007;111:47–53.
33. Federle MP, McGrath KM. Cystic neoplasms of the pancreas. Gastroenterol Clin North Am. 2007;36:365–76. ix.
34. Pais SA, Al-Haddad M, Mohamadnejad M, et al. EUS for pancreatic neuroendocrine tumors: a single-center, 11-year experience. Gastrointest Endosc. 2010;71:1185–93.
35. Baker MS, Knuth JL, DeWitt J, et al. Pancreatic cystic neuroendocrine tumors: preoperative diagnosis with endoscopic ultrasound and fine-needle immunocytology. J Gastrointest Surg. 2008;12:450–6.
36. Anderson MA, Carpenter S, Thompson NW, Nostrant TT, Elta GH, Scheiman JM. Endoscopic ultrasound is highly accurate and directs management in patients with neuroendocrine tumors of the pancreas. Am J Gastroenterol. 2000;95:2271–7.
37. Gouya H, Vignaux O, Augui J, et al. CT, endoscopic sonography, and a combined protocol for preoperative evaluation of pancreatic insulinomas. AJR Am J Roentgenol. 2003;181:987–92.
38. Ardengh JC, Rosenbaum P, Ganc AJ, et al. Role of EUS in the preoperative localization of insulinomas compared with spiral CT. Gastrointest Endosc. 2000;51:552–5.
39. Sotoudehmanesh R, Hedayat A, Shirazian N, et al. Endoscopic ultrasonography (EUS) in the localization of insulinoma. Endocrine. 2007;31:238–41.
40. Puli SR, Kalva N, Bechtold ML, et al. Diagnostic accuracy of endoscopic ultrasound in pancreatic neuroendocrine tumors: a systematic review and meta analysis. World J Gastroenterol. 2013;19:3678–84.
41. McLean AM, Fairclough PD. Endoscopic ultrasound in the localisation of pancreatic islet cell tumours. Best Pract Res Clin Endocrinol Metab. 2005;19:177–93.
42. Kann PH. The value of endoscopic ultrasound in localizing gastrinoma. Wien Klin Wochenschr. 2007;119:585–7.
43. Patel KK, Kim MK. Neuroendocrine tumors of the pancreas: endoscopic diagnosis. Curr Opin Gastroenterol. 2008;24:638–42.
44. Kann PH, Wirkus B, Keth A, Goitom K. Pitfalls in endosonographic imaging of suspected insulinomas: pancreatic nodules of unknown dignity. Eur J Endocrinol. 2003;148:531–4.
45. Kann PH, Ivan D, Pfutzner A, Forst T, Langer P, Schaefer S. Preoperative diagnosis of insulinoma: low body mass index, young age, and female gender are associated with negative imaging by endoscopic ultrasound. Eur J Endocrinol. 2007;157:209–13.
46. Klapman JB, Logrono R, Dye CE, Waxman I. Clinical impact of on-site cytopathology interpretation on endoscopic ultrasound-guided fine needle aspiration. Am J Gastroenterol. 2003;98:1289–94.
47. Alsohaibani F, Girgis S, Sandha GS. Does onsite cytotechnology evaluation improve the accuracy of endoscopic ultrasound-guided fine-needle aspiration biopsy? Can J Gastroenterol. 2009;23:26–30.
48. LeBlanc JK, Ciaccia D, Al-Assi MT, et al. Optimal number of EUS-guided fine needle passes needed to obtain a correct diagnosis. Gastrointest Endosc. 2004;59:475–81.

49. Erickson RA, Sayage-Rabie L, Beissner RS. Factors predicting the number of EUS-guided fine-needle passes for diagnosis of pancreatic malignancies. Gastrointest Endosc. 2000;51:184–90.
50. Chang F, Chandra A, Culora G, Mahadeva U, Meenan J, Herbert A. Cytologic diagnosis of pancreatic endocrine tumors by endoscopic ultrasound-guided fine-needle aspiration: a review. Diagn Cytopathol. 2006;34:649–58.
51. Chang F, Vu C, Chandra A, Meenan J, Herbert A. Endoscopic ultrasound-guided fine needle aspiration cytology of pancreatic neuroendocrine tumours: cytomorphological and immunocytochemical evaluation. Cytopathology. 2006;17:10–7.
52. Pais SMK, Leblanc J, et al. Utility of EUSFNA in the diagnosis of pancreatic neuroendocrine tumors: correlation with histopathology in 76 patients. Gastrointest Endosc. 2007;65:AB304.
53. Atiq M, Bhutani MS, Bektas M, et al. EUS-FNA for pancreatic neuroendocrine tumors: a tertiary cancer center experience. Dig Dis Sci. 2012;57:791–800.
54. Wittmann J, Kocjan G, Sgouros SN, Deheragoda M, Pereira SP. Endoscopic ultrasound-guided tissue sampling by combined fine needle aspiration and trucut needle biopsy: a prospective study. Cytopathology. 2006;17:27–33.
55. Varadarajulu S, Fraig M, Schmulewitz N, et al. Comparison of EUS-guided 19-gauge Trucut needle biopsy with EUS-guided fine-needle aspiration. Endoscopy. 2004;36:397–401.
56. Al-Haddad M, Gill KR, Raimondo M, et al. Safety and efficacy of cytology brushings versus standard fine-needle aspiration in evaluating cystic pancreatic lesions: a controlled study. Endoscopy. 2010;42:127–32.
57. Al-Haddad M, Raimondo M, Woodward T, et al. Safety and efficacy of cytology brushings versus standard FNA in evaluating cystic lesions of the pancreas: a pilot study. Gastrointest Endosc. 2007;65:894–8.
58. Nodit L, McGrath KM, Zahid M, et al. Endoscopic ultrasound-guided fine needle aspirate microsatellite loss analysis and pancreatic endocrine tumor outcome. Clin Gastroenterol Hepatol. 2006;4:1474–8.
59. Piani C, Franchi GM, Cappelletti C, et al. Cytological Ki-67 in pancreatic endocrine tumours: an opportunity for pre-operative grading. Endocr Relat Cancer. 2008;15:175–81.
60. Thomas-Marques L, Murat A, Delemer B, et al. Prospective endoscopic ultrasonographic evaluation of the frequency of nonfunctioning pancreaticoduodenal endocrine tumors in patients with multiple endocrine neoplasia type 1. Am J Gastroenterol. 2006;101:266–73.
61. Kann PH, Kann B, Fassbender WJ, Forst T, Bartsch DK, Langer P. Small neuroendocrine pancreatic tumors in multiple endocrine neoplasia type 1 (MEN1): least significant change of tumor diameter as determined by endoscopic ultrasound (EUS) imaging. Exp Clin Endocrinol Diabetes. 2006;114:361–5.
62. Lee LC, Grant CS, Salomao DR, et al. Small, nonfunctioning, asymptomatic pancreatic neuroendocrine tumors (PNETs): role for nonoperative management. Surgery. 2012;152:965–74.
63. Alsohaibani F, Bigam D, Kneteman N, Shapiro AM, Sandha GS. The impact of preoperative endoscopic ultrasound on the surgical management of pancreatic neuroendocrine tumours. Can J Gastroenterol. 2008;22:817–20.
64. Lewis MA, Thompson GB, Young Jr WF. Preoperative assessment of the pancreas in multiple endocrine neoplasia type 1. World J Surg. 2012;36:1375–81.
65. Zhang T, Mu Y, Qu L, et al. Accurate combined preoperative localization of insulinomas aid the choice for enucleation: a single institution experience over 25 years. Hepatogastroenterology. 2012;59:1282–5.
66. Varma V, Tariciotti L, Coldham C, Taniere P, Buckels JA, Bramhall SR. Preoperative localisation and surgical management of insulinoma: single centre experience. Dig Surg. 2011;28:63–73.
67. Wong M, Isa SH, Zahiah M, Azmi KN. Intraoperative ultrasound with palpation is still superior to intra-arterial calcium stimulation test in localising insulinoma. World J Surg. 2007;31:586–92.
68. Gress FG, Barawi M, Kim D, Grendell JH. Preoperative localization of a neuroendocrine tumor of the pancreas with EUS-guided fine needle tattooing. Gastrointest Endosc. 2002;55:594–7.

69. Zografos GN, Stathopoulou A, Mitropapas G, et al. Preoperative imaging and localization of small sized insulinoma with EUS-guided fine needle tattooing: a case report. Hormones. 2005;4:111–6.
70. Newman NA, Lennon AM, Edil BH, et al. Preoperative endoscopic tattooing of pancreatic body and tail lesions decreases operative time for laparoscopic distal pancreatectomy. Surgery. 2010;148:371–7.
71. Law JK, Singh VK, Khashab MA, et al. Endoscopic ultrasound (EUS)-guided fiducial placement allows localization of small neuroendocrine tumors during parenchymal-sparing pancreatic surgery. Surg Endosc. 2013;27:3921–6.
72. Saftoiu A, Dietrich CF, Vilmann P. Contrast-enhanced harmonic endoscopic ultrasound. Endoscopy. 2012;44:612–7.
73. Fusaroli P, Spada A, Mancino MG, Caletti G. Contrast harmonic echo-endoscopic ultrasound improves accuracy in diagnosis of solid pancreatic masses. Clin Gastroenterol Hepatol. 2010;8:629–34. e1–2.
74. Kitano M, Kudo M, Yamao K, et al. Characterization of small solid tumors in the pancreas: the value of contrast-enhanced harmonic endoscopic ultrasonography. Am J Gastroenterol. 2012;107:303–10.
75. Itokawa F, Itoi T, Sofuni A, et al. EUS elastography combined with the strain ratio of tissue elasticity for diagnosis of solid pancreatic masses. J Gastroenterol. 2011;46:843–53.
76. Iglesias-Garcia J, Larino-Noia J, Abdulkader I, Forteza J, Dominguez-Munoz JE. Quantitative endoscopic ultrasound elastography: an accurate method for the differentiation of solid pancreatic masses. Gastroenterology. 2010;139:1172–80.

Chapter 8
Endoscopic Approaches to Treatment of Pancreatic Neuroendocrine Neoplasms

Amit Raina and Vinay Chandrasekhara

Endoscopic therapies targeting pancreatic neuroendocrine tumors (PNETs) are not considered standard of care. This is especially true for patients with localized and potentially curable disease. On the other hand, endoscopic guided therapies, to debulk the tumor and/or to control symptoms, have been offered to patients with either metastatic disease or those who are poor surgical candidates [1, 2]. Various endoscopic ultrasound (EUS)-guided local ablation therapies such as radiofrequency ablation (RFA), photodynamic therapy, and brachytherapy are some of the other modalities that have been evaluated or are under investigation for the treatment of PNETs [2–5]. EUS has also been used to deliver fiducials within or adjacent to small PNETs to facilitate visualization of these small lesions at the time of parenchymal-sparing pancreatic surgery [6].

Endoscopic interventions have a better defined role in the management of synchronous gastric or duodenal neuroendocrine tumors that are often encountered in certain individuals with PNETs, such as those with MEN-I syndrome. Endoscopic techniques offer curative or palliative management of these subepithelial gastrointestinal lesions. Endoscopic modalities that are often used include endoscopic band ligation (EBL), endoscopic mucosal resection, and endoscopic submucosal dissection [5, 7, 8].

In the following paragraphs, we have summarized the literature on endoscopic-based therapies that have been offered to patients with PNETs and associated gastroenteropancreatic neuroendocrine neoplasms (GEP-NETs).

A. Raina, M.D.
Gastroenterology Division, East Carolina University, Greenville, NC, USA

V. Chandrasekhara, M.D. (✉)
Gastroenterology Division, University of Pennsylvania Health System,
1 Convention Avenue, 9 Penn Tower, Philadelphia, PA, USA
e-mail: Vinay.Chandrasekhara@uphs.upenn.edu

J.R. Pisegna (ed.), *Management of Pancreatic Neuroendocrine Tumors*,
DOI 10.1007/978-1-4939-1798-3_8

8.1 Gastrinomas

The majority of gastrinomas (approximately 70 %) are sporadic and remaining 30 % are associated with MEN-I [9]. The majority of the sporadic gastrinomas (60 %) and MEN-I-associated gastrinomas (90 %) arise from the duodenum, while the remaining are localized to pancreas or the adjacent lymph nodes [10]. Duodenal gastrinomas are typically small and multifocal, especially in patients with MEN-1. Patients with sporadic gastrinomas without obvious liver metastasis typically undergo surgical intervention. However, patients with MEN-1-associated gastrinomas are typically not offered surgical resection, even in the absence of liver metastasis, due to poor operative cure rates [11, 12]. Endoscopic resection techniques have been offered to patients with duodenal lesions for reducing the disease burden and in cases with isolated duodenal lesions, potentially offering a cure. Endoscopic resection may be curative in highly selected patients with duodenal neuroendocrine tumors less than 20 mm in diameter, localized within the submucosal layer as confirmed by a careful EUS examination, and without obvious metastatic disease [13, 14]. A report by Lee et al. highlighted a case of a functional duodenal gastrinoma that was successfully resected by EBL [15]. This patient had an 8 mm submucosal lesion in the second portion of the duodenum associated with an elevated gastrin level. Cross-sectional imaging did not detect any metastatic disease. EBL was performed using a standard endoscope with a commercially available band ligation kit. A transparent cap with bands was attached to tip of the endoscope and advanced to the target lesion. The cap was placed over the lesion, maximum suction applied, and the band was released around the base. Subsequent snare resection was not performed. Follow-up endoscopy demonstrated sloughing of the lesion. Biopsies from the scarred tissue showed no remnant tumor. Post-procedure serum gastrin levels declined after resection.

8.2 Insulinoma

Pancreatic insulinomas are usually small in size and present with recurrent hypoglycemic symptoms [16]. EUS allows high-resolution imaging of the pancreas and can detect small hypoechoic masses in the pancreas. Although pancreatic surgery is considered a first-line approach for insulinoma treatment, a subset of patients are not suitable for pancreatic surgery because of poor surgical candidacy or comorbid illness [17]. A number of endoscopically delivered techniques have been reported both in animal models and in human subjects that offer the option of reducing the tumor burden and improving symptoms in such patients, including RFA and alcohol ablation.

8.2.1 Radiofrequency Ablation

Goldberg et al. (1999) performed a study on the feasibility and the safety of EUS-guided RFA in the porcine pancreas [18]. RFA was applied to normal pancreatic tissue in 13 anesthetized Yorkshire pigs with specially modified 19-gauge needle electrodes. Subsequent laboratory, imaging, and histological evaluations of these pigs confirmed the safety and efficacy of delivering RFA treatment within the pancreatic parenchyma. With imaging and pathologic examination, the authors documented that 8–10 mm of coagulation necrosis was induced around the electrode. Recent animal studies by Kim et al. and Gaidhane et al. have confirmed the safety and feasibility of using RFA endoscopic therapy in porcine pancreas [3, 19]. On review of literature, only one case of percutaneous RFA of pancreatic tail gastrinomas was found [20]. However, given the safety of this procedure, as has been validated by recent animal studies, RFA may find a role in management of selected patients with PNETs who are deemed poor surgical candidates.

8.2.2 Alcohol Ablation

EUS-guided delivering of alcohol for ablation of solid pancreatic tumors has been reported by multiple authors. Jurgensen et al. reported successful EUS-guided ablation of PNET by ethanol injection [1]. The authors achieved complete resolution based on clinical, morphologic, and biochemical data. Deprez et al. reported successful EUS-guided injection of 5 mL of 98 % ethanol in the pancreatic tumor after endoprosthetic stenting of the biliary and pancreatic ducts, for a pancreatic head insulinoma [21]. This case was complicated by an asymptomatic elevation of pancreatic enzymes for 2 days as well as a hematoma and ulceration of the duodenal wall. Complete normalization of pancreatic head morphology was confirmed by imaging at 3 months after the intervention and the patient remained asymptomatic and normoglycemic more than 2 years after the procedure. The technique of introducing alcohol into pancreatic parenchyma appears to be safe, as illustrated by the above cases and also by larger studies that have studied the use of alcohol to ablate pancreatic cystic lesions in poor surgical candidates [22, 23]. However, alcohol ablation therapy is still considered investigational, and the standards for the type of injection needle, safe target area within tumor mass, and the adequate amount of alcohol to achieve successful ablation without causing significant pancreatitis are yet to be defined.

8.3 Somatostatinoma

Somatostatinomas are rare NET of the GI tract, commonly found in the pancreas head and the periampullary region. In contrast to its pancreatic counterpart, the duodenal somatostatinoma is frequently associated with von Recklinghausen disease and is very rarely associated with a clinically relevant "somatostatin syndrome." Endoscopic resection can be performed for small tumors <20 mm in diameter if there is no evidence of infiltration of the muscularis propria or local lymph node metastasis. A prior echoendoscopy (EUS) is vital for determining feasibility for an endoscopic approach. Marques et al. recently reported endoscopic submucosal dissection of solitary duodenal somatostatinoma [24]. Echoendoscopy was used to confirm feasibility of such resection by demonstrating a lack of infiltration into the muscularis propria and without obvious lymph node spread. Following the mucosal dissection, histology confirmed the diagnosis and confirmed that the margins were free of tumor.

8.4 Subepithelial Lesions of the Stomach and the Duodenum Associated with PNETS

8.4.1 Gastric

Gastric carcinoid tumors are divided into three types. Type 1 gastric carcinoid accounts for 70–85 % of all gastric carcinoids and is associated with chronic atrophic gastritis. Type 1 lesions are often multifocal and usually small (1 cm or less) with a low malignant potential. Type 2 gastric carcinoid accounts for 5–10 % of all gastric carcinoids and is associated with Zollinger-Ellison syndrome with or without MEN-1 syndrome. Similar to type 1 gastric carcinoid, type 2 lesions are multicentric, small, with an indolent clinical behavior. Type 2 gastric carcinoids are encountered in 15–50 % of patients with MEN-1 [25]. Up to 30 % of these type 2 gastric carcinoids may metastasize regionally to lymph nodes [10]. Given the low risk of metastasis with type 1 and type 2 gastric carcinoids, endoscopic resection often provides adequate therapy, particularly for lesions smaller than 1–2 cm in size [13]. EUS is valuable for this approach and helps to determine the depth of involvement and provides an accurate means for determining the presence or absence of lymph node metastasis. Endoscopic resection is typically performed using standard snare resection techniques. After endoscopic resection, surveillance with endoscopy is recommended every 6–12 months to confirm clearance. However, some patients often continue to exhibit mucosal changes and hyperplasia of enterochromaffin-like cells (ECL) due to sustained hypergastrinemia.

Type 3 gastric carcinoids account for 15–25 % of all gastric carcinoids and are not associated with elevated gastrin levels [26]. These lesions portend a higher risk of lymph node or hepatic metastasis and often require surgical resection, particularly for lesions larger than 2 cm.

8.4.2 Duodenum

Duodenal neuroendocrine tumors include gastrinomas, somatostatinomas, nonfunctional NETs, gangliocytic paragangliomas, and poorly differentiated neuroendocrine carcinomas [27]. Duodenal somatostatinomas show a preference for the periampullary region and are often seen in patients with neurofibromatosis 1 (von Recklinghausen's disease). Sporadic duodenal NETs are usually solitary, in contrast to multifocal NETs seen in patients with MEN-1 [27]. Similar to gastrinomas, if the muscularis is invaded, metastasis to regional nodes is frequent. Duodenal NETs that are less than 1 cm and not associated with Zollinger-Ellison syndrome rarely develop metastases [28]. It has been recommended that endoscopic treatment or excision is likely to be adequate for non-metastatic duodenal NETs less than 1 cm, provided they are limited to the submucosa. As with gastric lesions, EUS is helpful in assessing for endoscopic resectability of these lesions [13].

References

1. Jurgensen C, Schuppan D, Neser F, et al. EUS-guided alcohol ablation of an insulinoma. Gastrointest Endosc. 2006;63:1059–62.
2. Seo DW. EUS-guided antitumor therapy for pancreatic tumors. Gut Liver. 2010;4 Suppl 1:S76–81.
3. Gaidhane M, Smith I, Ellen K, et al. Endoscopic ultrasound-guided radiofrequency ablation (EUS-RFA) of the pancreas in a porcine model. Gastroenterol Res Pract. 2012;2012:431451.
4. Scott A, Hinwood D, Donnelly R. Radio-frequency ablation for symptom control in a patient with metastatic pancreatic insulinoma. Clin Endocrinol (Oxf). 2002;56:557–9.
5. Varas MJ, Gornals JB, Pons C, et al. Usefulness of endoscopic ultrasonography (EUS) for selecting carcinoid tumors as candidates to endoscopic resection. Rev Esp Enferm Dig. 2010;102:577–82.
6. Law JK, Singh VK, Khashab MA, et al. Endoscopic ultrasound (EUS)-guided fiducial placement allows localization of small neuroendocrine tumors during parenchymal-sparing pancreatic surgery. Surg Endosc. 2013;27:3921–6.
7. Chen WF, Zhou PH, Li QL, et al. Clinical impact of endoscopic submucosal dissection for gastric neuroendocrine tumors: a retrospective study from mainland of China. Scientific World J. 2012;2012:869769.
8. Gomez V, Groce JR, Xaio SY, et al. Band ligation resection of duodenal carcinoid (with video). Gastrointest Endosc. 2007;66:397. discussion 398.
9. Metz DC, Jensen RT. Gastrointestinal neuroendocrine tumors: pancreatic endocrine tumors. Gastroenterology. 2008;135:1469–92.
10. Frilling A, Akerstrom G, Falconi M, et al. Neuroendocrine tumor disease: an evolving landscape. Endocr Relat Cancer. 2012;19:R163–85.
11. Imamura M, Komoto I, Ota S, et al. Biochemically curative surgery for gastrinoma in multiple endocrine neoplasia type 1 patients. World J Gastroenterol. 2011;17:1343–53.
12. Thakker RV, Newey PJ, Walls GV, et al. Clinical practice guidelines for multiple endocrine neoplasia type 1 (MEN1). J Clin Endocrinol Metab. 2012;97:2990–3011.
13. Scherubl H, Jensen RT, Cadiot G, et al. Management of early gastrointestinal neuroendocrine neoplasms. World J Gastrointest Endosc. 2011;3:133–9.
14. Dalenback J, Havel G. Local endoscopic removal of duodenal carcinoid tumors. Endoscopy. 2004;36:651–5.
15. Lee SH, Hong YS, Lee JM, et al. Duodenal gastrinoma treated with endoscopic band ligation. Gastrointest Endosc. 2009;69:964–7.
16. Milan SA, Yeo CJ. Neuroendocrine tumors of the pancreas. Curr Opin Oncol. 2012; 24:46–55.
17. DiNorcia J, Lee MK, Reavey PL, et al. One hundred thirty resections for pancreatic neuroendocrine tumor: evaluating the impact of minimally invasive and parenchyma-sparing techniques. J Gastrointest Surg. 2010;14:1536–46.
18. Goldberg SN, Mallery S, Gazelle GS, et al. EUS-guided radiofrequency ablation in the pancreas: results in a porcine model. Gastrointest Endosc. 1999;50:392–401.

19. Kim HJ, Seo DW, Hassanuddin A, et al. EUS-guided radiofrequency ablation of the porcine pancreas. Gastrointest Endosc. 2012;76:1039–43.
20. Wu PH, Pan CC, Huang ZL, et al. Percutaneous radiofrequency ablation approach through the spleen: initial case report for pancreatic tail gastrinoma. Chin J Cancer. 2010;29:836–41.
21. Deprez PH, Claessens A, Borbath I, et al. Successful endoscopic ultrasound-guided ethanol ablation of a sporadic insulinoma. Acta Gastroenterol Belg. 2008;71:333–7.
22. DiMaio CJ, DeWitt JM, Brugge WR. Ablation of pancreatic cystic lesions: the use of multiple endoscopic ultrasound-guided ethanol lavage sessions. Pancreas. 2011;40:664–8.
23. DeWitt J, DiMaio CJ, Brugge WR. Long-term follow-up of pancreatic cysts that resolve radiologically after EUS-guided ethanol ablation. Gastrointest Endosc. 2010;72:862–6.
24. Marques I, Ribeiro MD, Pimentel-Nunes P, et al. Endoscopic submucosal dissection of solitary duodenal somatostatinoma (with video). Gastrointest Endosc. 2012;76:693–4.
25. Norton JA, Melcher ML, Gibril F, et al. Gastric carcinoid tumors in multiple endocrine neoplasia-1 patients with Zollinger-Ellison syndrome can be symptomatic, demonstrate aggressive growth, and require surgical treatment. Surgery. 2004;136:1267–74.
26. Nikou GC, Angelopoulos TP. Current concepts on gastric carcinoid tumors. Gastroenterol Res Pract. 2012;2012:287825.
27. Hoffmann KM, Furukawa M, Jensen RT. Duodenal neuroendocrine tumors: classification, functional syndromes, diagnosis and medical treatment. Best Pract Res. 2005;19:675–97.
28. Witzigmann HLC, Geissler F, et al. Neuroendocrine tumours of the duodenum. Clinical aspects, pathomorphology and therapy. Langenbecks Arch Surg. 2002;386:525–33.

Chapter 9
Surgical Approaches to Pancreatic Neuroendocrine Tumors

James X. Wu and F. Charles Brunicardi

9.1 Introduction

Surgical resection remains the mainstay of treatment for pancreatic neuroendocrine tumors (PNETs). Complete resection remains the only curative intervention. Nonetheless, even systemic disease often can be treated with cytoreductive surgery and/or interventional ablation techniques. The benefit of surgical intervention and the best procedure depends on the histologic subtype, location of the primary tumor, presence of metastasis, and whether patients have a multiple endocrine neoplasia type I (MEN-1) or von Hippel-Lindau syndrome. The surgical approach to nonfunctional PNETs, insulinomas, gastrinomas, and less common functional PNETs is covered, followed by a review of postsurgical complications and current controversies.

J.X. Wu, M.D.
Ronald Reagan UCLA Medical Center, 757 Westwood Plaza,
Mail Room B711, Los Angeles, CA 90095, USA
e-mail: jameswu@mednet.ucla.edu

F.C. Brunicardi, M.D., F.A.C.S. (✉)
Ronald Reagan UCLA Medical Center, 757 Westwood Plaza,
Mail Room B711, Los Angeles, CA 90095, USA

UCLA Medical Center, Santa Monica, CA, USA
e-mail: CBrunicardi@mednet.ucla.edu

J.R. Pisegna (ed.), *Management of Pancreatic Neuroendocrine Tumors*,
DOI 10.1007/978-1-4939-1798-3_9

9.2 Nonfunctional Pancreatic Neuroendocrine Tumors

9.2.1 Preoperative Assessment and Imaging

Nonfunctional PNETs often present with vague symptoms, such as nonspecific abdominal pain, early satiety, or weight loss; locally advanced lesions can present with bowel obstruction or obstructive jaundice. Many are incidentally discovered on imaging. Serum chromogranin A (CgA) levels can be elevated with nonfunctional PNETs. CgA levels should be drawn at baseline to monitor disease progression and response to treatment; however, it is not an appropriate screening test. Serum CgA can be elevated due to other causes including proton pump inhibitor use, atrophic gastritis, or liver or renal failure. If CgA testing is indeterminate, pancreatic polypeptide is also elevated in 50–80 % of PNETs [1]. Finally, every preoperative workup should include a detailed family history to detect MEN-1 and VHL, which should lead to MEN-1 gene or VHL gene testing, respectively.

There is no established imaging algorithm for PNETs. As mentioned above, pancreatic lesions are often discovered incidentally on cross-sectional imaging. Diagnostic imaging for suspected PNETs should begin with a multiphase abdominal CT scan with intravenous contrast using a pancreatic protocol. PNETs enhance with contrast in the arterial phase and washout in the delayed venous phase. If suspicion for PNET is high, initial CT scan can be combined with somatostatin receptor scintigraphy (SRS). SRS is the most sensitive test compared to CT, MRI, and US, however, although it is sensitive for tumor location, it does not give reliable information regarding tumor size [2]. After CT/SRS, indeterminate hepatic lesions can be better evaluated by MRI. Lesions >2 cm in size should undergo a thorough investigation for distant disease, as the risk of metastasis increases with tumor size (Fig. 9.1).

Once a pancreatic lesion is identified or suspicion is high despite nondiagnostic cross-sectional imaging, endoscopic ultrasound (EUS) is indicated. EUS can detect smaller or multifocal lesions, identify regional lymph nodes, and evaluate the pancreatic duct and vasculature for operative planning. Fine-needle aspiration should be performed during EUS to obtain a tissue diagnosis when the tumor is not resectable, as tissue diagnosis can guide therapy. EUS-FNA has a diagnostic yield of 90–93 % [3]. In resectable cases, India ink injection can also be performed at time of EUS to help localize the tumor intraoperatively. Finally, if imaging results are still inconclusive, F18-FDG-PET/CT has been reported to be useful in evaluating high-grade PNETs.

9.2.2 Surgical Approach to Localized Nonfunctional PNETs

Surgery is the only curative therapy, and localized disease should be treated with intent to cure. Enucleation can be considered in small, low-grade, solitary PNETs (<2 cm) in younger patients if confirmed on EUS not to involve the main pancreatic duct,

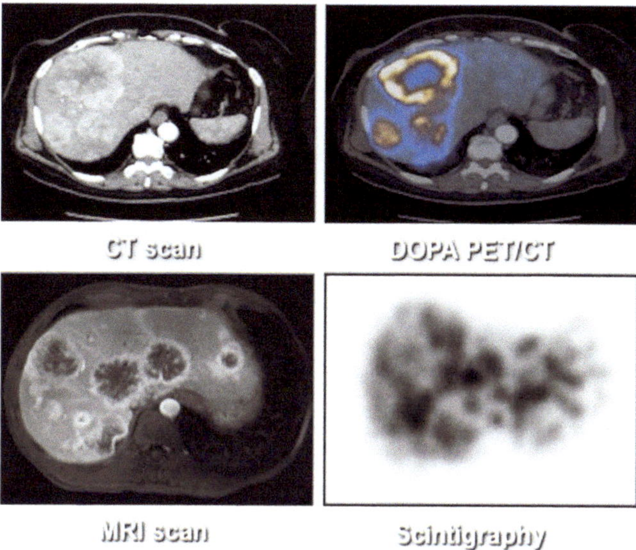

Fig. 9.1 Hepatic metastases seen on various imaging modalities from pancreatic neuroendocrine tumor

but partial pancreatectomy is preferred over enucleation [4]. Lesions within the pancreatic head should undergo Whipple procedure (pancreaticoduodenectomy), and lesions in the body and tail should undergo distal pancreatectomy. Whipple procedures remove the gallbladder, duodenum, and proximal pancreas, which requires reconstruction of the anastomosis between the common bile duct and pancreatic duct with the small intestine. Distal pancreatectomy often is accompanied by splenectomy, and those patients should receive appropriate vaccination against encapsulated bacteria. Select patients with diffuse disease can also undergo total pancreatectomy, but the benefit has not been demonstrated. Finally, central pancreatectomy has been largely abandoned due to high postoperative morbidity, but still considered by some centers in special circumstances in young patients [5]. All the above procedures can be done open or laparoscopically; the choice should be based on the experience of individual centers (Fig. 9.2).

Following surgical resection, 5-year survival rates for local disease are 77–93 % [6, 7]. For locally advanced disease, the 5-year survival is 46 % after resection [7].

For locally advanced disease without metastases, if more than 90 % of disease can be resected, cytoreductive surgery should be pursued [4]. If patients presented with obstructive symptoms, palliative bypass surgery can also be performed at this time.

Patients that have MEN-1 and VHL often have multifocal disease. Some surgeons may choose to perform distal pancreatectomy followed by enucleation of tumors located in the head of the pancreas. In VHL, one series recommends surveillance of lesions <1 cm, resection of lesions >2 cm when located in the head of the pancreas,

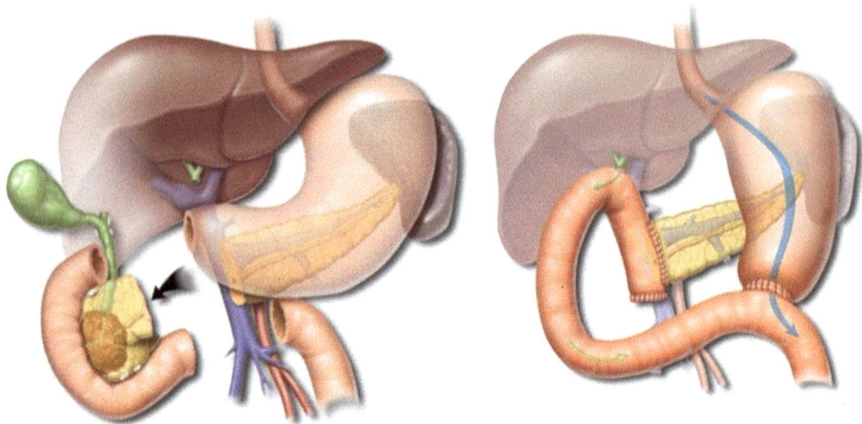

Fig. 9.2 Pancreaticoduodenectomy. From Schwartz Principles of Surgery, 9th edition

and resection of lesions that are >3 cm that are increasing in size. If surgery will be pursued, the procedure should always include intraoperative ultrasound and enucleation when possible to spare normal tissue [8].

9.2.3 Surgical Approach to Nonfunctional PNETs with Liver Metastases

The goal of surgical treatment of hepatic metastases is complete resection, but surgery can still be attempted if >90 % cytoreduction can be achieved. Hepatic resection is accomplished by wedge resections, which follow nonanatomic lines of dissection, or left versus right hepatectomy or hepatic segmentectomies, which follow anatomic lines of dissection. Wedge resections preserve more liver tissue but increase risk of bleeding. The choice of procedure should spare as much normal liver tissue as possible, while aiming for complete resection of disease. The major limiting factor is preserving enough liver function. In patients with normal liver function, the remnant liver needs to be 20–30 % of the original liver volume [9]. For patients with preexisting liver disease, patients should undergo volumetric CT scan and liver function testing to determine the relative decrease in their liver function per volume.

Patients that received hepatic resection have the same rate of disease-free survival as patients with localized disease, strongly suggesting a benefit from surgical therapy [10]. After complete resection, 5-year survival rates are 56–73 % [6, 11–13]. Even with patients that receive a complete resection, disease-free survival at 5 years is only about 10 % [6]. Rates of recurrence following >90 % resection remain high, with only 3.5 % of patients free of disease at 5 years, but resection is still associated with increased survival [6, 14].

The timing of hepatic resection relative to the pancreatic resection appears to favor simultaneous resection. A large series from the Mayo Clinic and Johns Hopkins Hospital showed simultaneous pancreatic and hepatic resection is associated with decreased morbidity, and reduces risk of liver abscess [15]. However, there may be significant selection bias, where patients that could not tolerate a simultaneous procedure were less healthy at baseline. Ultimately, timing of procedures is left to the surgeon's judgment weighing the patient's fitness for a single prolonged procedure.

When hepatic metastases are unresectable with surgery alone due to the number of liver lesions or large tumor size, ablation can be used alone or in conjunction with surgery. Adequate cytoreduction can be achieved by combining liver surgery with ablation techniques, either intraoperatively or percutaneously at a later time. Ablation techniques include cryoablation, ethanol injection, and radiofrequency ablation. Cryoablation and ethanol injection both are performed with intraoperative ultrasound guidance, and able to achieve complete response in small tumors. RFA is now more commonly used, which uses a high-frequency current to generate heat. RFA of hepatic neuroendocrine tumor metastases is associated with low morbidity and achieves significant symptom relief in 80 % of patients as well as no disease progression in 40 % [16].

Bulky, unresectable liver disease can also be treated with arterial embolization or liver transplantation. Embolization of hepatic artery preferentially targets tumor cells, given that hepatic parenchyma depends on portal venous blood flow. Hepatic artery embolization can either be done with "bland" particles or cytotoxic chemotherapy agents. In transcatheter arterial chemoembolization (TACE), the hepatic artery supplying blood to area with greatest tumor burden is catheterized and a chemotherapeutic agent such as streptozotocin is infused. For PNETs, chemoembolization results in improved survival over bland embolization [17]. Alternatively, liver transplantation can be considered. Criteria for liver transplantation for neuroendocrine tumors with liver metastases are age <50 years, Ki-67 index low, positivity for cadherin on immunohistochemistry, and hepatic tumor involvement less than 50 % [18]. The benefit of liver transplantation for PNETs has yet to be fully characterized.

9.3 Insulinoma

9.3.1 Preoperative Assessment and Imaging

The classical symptoms of insulinomas are described in Whipple's triad: symptomatic fasting hypoglycemia, documented serum glucose <50 mg/dL, and symptomatic relief with glucose supplementation. Serum C-peptide should also be drawn to rule out factitious hypoglycemia. A detailed family history should also be obtained, given that approximately 10 % of insulinomas are associated with MEN-1 [19].

Insulinomas can be visualized with multiphase CT scan of the abdomen with intravenous contrast. Patients should also receive EUS, which has increased sensitivity for lesions compared to CT [19]. SRS is less useful, but can help detect metastatic or occult disease when it is not found on CT or EUS, but only has a sensitivity of 60 % [20]. Overall, current imaging techniques have a 98 % sensitivity for localizing insulinomas [19].

Even if all attempts to localize the tumor fail with preoperative imaging, it is reasonable to proceed to surgery if there is enough supporting biochemical evidence consistent with an insulinoma. If exploratory laparotomy is performed for insulinoma, patients should undergo distal pancreatectomy, manual palpation of the pancreas, and intraoperative ultrasound.

9.3.2 Surgical Approach

Due to the relatively benign nature of insulinomas, small, localized that do not involve the main pancreatic duct can be treated with enucleation. Otherwise, lesions can undergo appropriate partial pancreatectomy based upon the location of the disease: Whipple for pancreatic head and uncinate lesions and distal pancreatectomy for pancreatic body and tail lesions. During the operation the pancreas should be manually palpated to assess for additional lesions. Lesions can be evaluated with intraoperative ultrasound to delineate the relationship between the tumor and duct. Following resection of localized disease, frozen sections should be sent to confirm tumor-negative surgical margins. Hepatic metastases should be approached similarly to nonfunctional PNETs.

Following resection, overall 5- and 10-year survival is 97 % and 86 %, respectively; 90 % of patients remain disease-free at 5 years after surgery [19].

Surgeons and anesthesiologists should also be mindful of potential insulin release during the operation. Anesthesiologists should remain vigilant with regard to drops in blood sugar during manipulation of the pancreas.

9.4 Gastrinoma

9.4.1 Preoperative Assessment and Imaging

Gastrin-secreting tumors, usually complain of peptic ulcer disease that may be refractory to antacids and can also have generalized abdominal pain, esophagitis, and/or diarrhea. Fasting serum gastrin >1,000 pg/mL is highly suggestive of gastrinoma, and a secretin stimulation test can help as well. Prior to serum gastrin measurements, proton pump inhibitors and histamine type 2 blockers should be stopped for 1 week or 2 days, respectively. Again, family history of MEN-1 or VHL should be elucidated as up to 25 % of gastrinomas can be part of MEN-1 syndrome.

Localization should be performed with SRS and CT scan, which has 100 % combined sensitivity [21]. The majority of gastrinomas (70–90 %) will be found in Passaro's triangle, formed by where the cystic duct meets the common bile duct, 2nd–3rd portion of the duodenum, and neck of the pancreas. Following SRS, EUS should be performed to assess for subcentimeter lesions in the pancreas or duodenal wall.

9.4.2 *Surgical Approach*

Similar to insulinomas, small, localized gastrinomas that do not involve the main pancreatic duct can be enucleated; otherwise, pancreatic resection can be performed. For occult gastrinomas, patients can undergo highly selective vagotomy. This procedure can decrease PPI use. The 15-year survival rate for localized gastrinomas is 80 %.

Even in patients with MEN-1 syndrome, 77 % of patients that underwent pancreatic resection were eugastremic [22]. However, the surgical management of patients with MEN-1 or VHL is controversial. Per published 2012 consensus guidelines on management of patients with MEN-1, surgery for patients with MEN-1 should be individualized, though most centers perform surgery only for gastrinomas >2 cm Whipple for gastrinoma should be reserved for specialty centers [23]. Patients with MEN-1 and metastatic gastrinoma do not benefit from debulking surgery, but may be candidates for cytoreductive ablation. The 5-year survival rate even in the presence of hepatic metastases is 20–50 %.

9.5 Uncommon Functional PNETs

9.5.1 *VIPoma*

The most classical symptom of VIPoma is episodic watery diarrhea. Serial measurements of VIP are usually needed, given that basal levels fluctuate. These are mostly located in the distal pancreas. Resection should follow the same protocol as nonfunctional PNETs. For advanced disease, surgical debulking can help palliate symptoms.

9.5.2 *Glucagonoma*

The classic syndrome is dermatitis with diabetes. Necrolytic migratory erythema is commonly seen around the mouth, lower abdomen, perineum, and feet and believed to be due to low amino acids. Confirmatory laboratory testing involves measuring glucagon levels, which are usually >500 pg/mL. These also occur more often in the distal pancreas. Resection is similar to nonfunctional PNETs, and symptoms typically respond to debulking surgeries.

9.5.3 *Somatostatinoma*

These patients present with gallstones, diabetes, and steatorrhea. Confirmatory testing is serum somatostatin, usually >10 ng/mL. These occur more often in the proximal pancreas, commonly near the ampulla. Surgery should include cholecystectomy.

9.6 Common Postoperative Complications

Pancreatic resections are associated with a significant rate of morbidity. Almost one fifth of patients that undergo pancreaticoduodenectomy are readmitted within 30 days [24]. The Whipple procedure is associated with 48 % risk of postoperative complications, and distal pancreatectomy has a 12.5 % risk of complications [25].

Pancreatic leaks occur frequently following pancreatic resection. They are diagnosed by testing surgical drain fluid for amylase and/or lipase levels and by abdominal CT scan. Initial therapies for pancreatic leaks are conservative, as a majority are self-limited. Conservative management includes minimization of pancreatic output by making patients NPO or by using nasojejunal feeding and supportive care, and if the fistula is external, protective skin care is necessary. Somatostatin has not been effective in increasing fistula closure rate [26].

If conservative therapy fails, then endoscopic, percutaneous, or surgical treatments may be attempted. Endoscopic therapy includes placing a pancreatic stent so that pancreatic secretions will follow the path of least resistance into the duodenum, can also drain lesions if accessible. Surgical therapy is typically delayed for a minimum of 4–6 weeks to allow time for the fistula tract to fibrose.

Delayed gastric emptying also occurs after Whipple procedures, leading to nausea, vomiting, abdominal discomfort, and early satiety. Pylorus-preserving pancreaticoduodenectomy significantly increases rate of delayed gastric emptying [27]. This can be treated medically with erythromycin or metoclopramide.

Other surgical complications include biliary leaks, anastomotic leaks, hemorrhage, and superficial and deep space infections. Biliary leaks can be managed conservatively initially if surgical drains remain in place. Bilomas should be drained percutaneously to avoid infection. If these persist, they may require endoscopic intervention with biliary stent placement. Anastomotic leaks can present insidiously with isolated tachycardia initially, followed by increased pain or evidence of peritonitis on abdominal exam.

References

1. Ramage JK, Ahmed A, Ardill J, et al. Guidelines for the management of gastroenteropancreatic neuroendocrine (including carcinoid) tumours (NETs). Gut. 2012;61:6–32.
2. Sundin A, Garske U, Orlefors H. Nuclear imaging of neuroendocrine tumours. Best Pract Res Clin Endocrinol Metab. 2007;21:69–85.
3. Atiq M, Bhutani MS, Bektas M, et al. EUS-FNA for pancreatic neuroendocrine tumors: a tertiary cancer center experience. Dig Dis Sci. 2012;57:791–800.
4. Burns WR, Edil BH. Neuroendocrine pancreatic tumors: guidelines for management and update. Curr Treat Options Oncol. 2012;13:24–34.
5. Goudard Y, Gaujoux S, Dokmak S, et al. Reappraisal of central pancreatectomy a 12-year single-center experience. JAMA. 2014;149:357.
6. Cusati D, Zhang L, Harmsen WS, et al. Metastatic nonfunctioning pancreatic neuroendocrine carcinoma to liver: surgical treatment and outcomes. J Am Coll Surg. 2012;215:117–24. discussion 124-115.
7. Solorzano CC, Lee JE, Pisters PWT, et al. Nonfunctioning islet cell carcinoma of the pancreas: survival results in a contemporary series of 163 patients. Surgery. 2001;130:1078–85.
8. Libutti SK, Choyke PL, Bartlett DL, et al. Pancreatic neuroendocrine tumors associated with von Hippel Lindau disease: diagnostic and management recommendations. Surgery. 1998;124:1153–9.
9. Guglielmi A, Ruzzenente A, Conci S, et al. How much remnant is enough in liver resection? Dig Surg. 2012;29:6–17.
10. Kleine M, Schrem H, Vondran FWR, et al. Extended surgery for advanced pancreatic endocrine tumours. Br J Surg. 2012;99:88–94.
11. Dousset B, Saint-Marc O, Pitre J, et al. Metastatic endocrine tumors: medical treatment, surgical resection, or liver transplantation. World J Surg. 1996;20:908–15.
12. Chen H, Hardacre JM, Uzar A, et al. Isolated liver metastases from neuroendocrine tumors: does resection prolong survival? J Am Coll Surg. 1998;187:88–92.
13. Ellison TA, Wolfgang CL, Shi C, et al. A single institution's 26-year experience with nonfunctional pancreatic neuroendocrine tumors: a validation of current staging systems and a new prognostic nomogram. Ann Surg. 2014;259:204–12.
14. Fischer L, Kleeff J, Esposito I, et al. Clinical outcome and long-term survival in 118 consecutive patients with neuroendocrine tumours of the pancreas. Br J Surg. 2008;95:627–35.
15. De Jong MC, Farnell MB, Sclabas G, et al. Liver-directed therapy for hepatic metastases in patients undergoing pancreaticoduodenectomy: a dual-center analysis. Ann Surg. 2010; 252:142–8.
16. Berber E, Flesher N, Siperstein AE. Laparoscopic radiofrequency ablation of neuroendocrine liver metastases. World J Surg. 2002;26:985–90.
17. Gupta S, Johnson MM, Murthy R, et al. Hepatic arterial embolization and chemoembolization for the treatment of patients with metastatic neuroendocrine tumors. Cancer. 2005;104:1590–602.
18. Mazzaferro V, Pulvirenti A, Coppa J. Neuroendocrine tumors metastatic to the liver: how to select patients for liver transplantation? J Hepatol. 2007;47:460–6.
19. Nikfarjam M, Warshaw AL, Axelrod L, et al. Improved contemporary surgical management of insulinomas: a 25-year experience at the Massachusetts General Hospital. Ann Surg. 2008;247:165–72.
20. Proye C, Malvaux P, Pattou F, et al. Noninvasive imaging of insulinomas and gastrinomas with endoscopic ultrasonography and somatostatin receptor scintigraphy. Surgery. 1998;124:1134–43. discussion 1143-1134.
21. Atema JJ, Amri R, Busch OR, et al. Surgical treatment of gastrinomas: a single-centre experience. HPB (Oxford). 2012;14:833–8.
22. Tonelli F, Fratini G, Nesi G, et al. Pancreatectomy in multiple endocrine neoplasia type 1-related gastrinomas and pancreatic endocrine neoplasias. Ann Surg. 2006;244:61.

23. Thakker RV, Newey PJ, Walls GV, et al. Clinical practice guidelines for multiple endocrine neoplasia type 1 (MEN1). J Clin Endocrinol Metab. 2012;97:2990–3011.
24. Hyder O, Dodson RM, Nathan H, et al. Influence of patient, physician, and hospital factors on 30-day readmission following pancreatoduodenectomy in the United States. JAMA Surg. 2013;148:1095–102.
25. Kazanjian KK, Reber HA, Hines OJ. Resection of pancreatic neuroendocrine tumors: results of 70 cases. Arch Surg. 2006;141:765–9. discussion 769-770.
26. Gans SL, van Westreenen HL, Kiewiet JJ, et al. Systematic review and meta-analysis of somatostatin analogues for the treatment of pancreatic fistula. Br J Surg. 2012;99:754–60.
27. Yang C, Wu HS, Chen XL, et al. Pylorus-preserving versus pylorus-resecting pancreaticoduodenectomy for periampullary and pancreatic carcinoma: a meta-analysis. PLoS One. 2014;9:e90316.

Chapter 10
Radiotherapy and Radiopharmaceuticals for the Treatment of Pancreatic Neuroendocrine Tumors

Lowell B. Anthony and Partha Sinha

Gastroenteropancreatic neuroendocrine tumors (GEP-NETs) are typically slow growing tumors of the endocrine pancreas and are often functional. They express somatostatin receptors, and the feasibility of imaging such tumors using radioiodinated somatostatin analogs in 1989 by Krenning et al. [1] led to the exploration of the possibilities to not only develop further imaging agents but also to develop therapeutic agents.

These therapeutic agents are pharmaceutical products with a radioactive atom attached. The pharmaceutical, in this case somatostatin or its analog, allows specific targeting of the receptor-expressing cells. This technique of targeting radionuclide therapy via specific receptors has been termed peptide receptor radionuclide therapy (PRRT). This allows the radioactive atom tagged to the pharmaceutical to be at very close proximity or at times even inside the cell. This is of benefit as for radionuclide therapy to be effective; the radioactive atom has a therapeutic range of a few cell diameters; and the short range spares the normal cells not expressing the receptors. However, this limits effective therapy. Higher energy levels increase the therapeutic range but kill all cells within that range. Broad physical principles of radionuclide therapy have been discussed elsewhere [2]. For radiobiological reasons, beta emitters are thought to be more suitable for radionuclide therapy than gamma emitters. Alpha emitters have further theoretical advantages over beta emitters in treating micrometastases and being able to selectively deliver higher doses of radiation to smaller volumes.

L.B. Anthony, M.D., F.A.C.P. (✉)
Division of Medical Oncology, Markey Cancer Center, University of Kentucky, Lexington, KY 40536-0093, USA
e-mail: lowell.anthony@uky.edu

P. Sinha M.D.
Division of Nuclear Medicine, Department of Radiology, University of Kentucky, Lexington, KY 40536, USA

J.R. Pisegna (ed.), *Management of Pancreatic Neuroendocrine Tumors*,
DOI 10.1007/978-1-4939-1798-3_10

10.1 131I-MIBG

131I-Metaiodobenzylguanidine (MIBG) has been used in the treatment of neuroendocrine tumors, particularly neuroblastoma, pheochromocytoma, paragangliomas, and carcinoids. It has also been used to treat other neuroendocrine tumors such as GEP-NETs, though currently PRRT is the preferred approach to treat these [3, 4].

MIBG is a norepinephrine analog which is taken up into the tumor cells primarily by the active energy-dependent catecholamine reuptake system (type 1) and gets stored in the norepinephrine secretory granules. Much less uptake takes place by the energy-independent nonspecific diffusion process (type 2) [5].

A considerable number of pharmacologic products interfere with MIBG uptake [6, 7]. These include commonly used medications such as calcium channel blockers, salbutamol, phenylephrine, and ephedrine among others. To enable MIBG uptake, these medications should be withdrawn prior to MIBG administration. The exact length of withdrawal depends on the frequency of administration of these medications. Withdrawal for two dosage intervals is sufficient in most cases. Before the actual treatment with 131I-MIBG, avidity of the lesions to MIBG should be documented by imaging with 123I-MIBG. This will ensure uptake of the therapeutic dose of 131I-MIBG by the tumor cells. As presence of free radioiodine is inevitable in 131I-MIBG preparations, uptake of radioiodine by the thyroid should be blocked by oral potassium perchlorate 400 mg per day. This acts as a competitive inhibitor of the sodium iodide symporter. Similarly, potassium iodide solution drops (maximum dose 40 drops/day) taken orally can saturate the body with iodine preventing further thyroidal uptake of 131-I. Either of these should be taken starting the day before therapy and continuing for 10–15 days post-therapy. The European Association of Nuclear Medicine (EANM) recommends usage of both potassium perchlorate and iodine saturation [7].

Typical adult dose of 131IMIBG is 100–300 mCi (3.7–11.1 GBq) administered intravenously over a period of 45 min–4 h using a lead-shielded infusion system [7]. The prolonged infusion is necessary when carrier-added MIBG is used as it contains significant amounts of non-radiolabeled MIBG which can produce pharmacologic sympathomimetic effects. Heart rate and blood pressure should therefore be monitored. Patients may complain of acute nausea. Premedicating with antiemetics may be justified. Patients will need to be placed under radiation protection as per local applicable regulations and discharged accordingly. As myelosuppression is common, with nadir in 4–6 weeks, monitoring of blood counts every 2–3 weeks will be necessary [3]. As can be expected, myelotoxicity appears to be dose related. In a retrospective study by Castellani et al., 83 % of patients had no myelotoxicity and the remaining 17 % had mild toxicity when less than 150 mCi (5.6 GBq) dose was used. At doses above this, 50 % of patients developed toxicity, only 12.5 % of which were mild [8].

Symptomatic response has varied between 44 and 73 %, with biochemical response varying between 15 and 50 % [9, 10]. Radiological response rates are less impressive with response rates less than 30 %. However, a retrospective study in 98 patients has demonstrated significant survival benefits related to symptomatic response but not to biochemical or radiological response. The same study demonstrated longer survival for those receiving high dose defined as more than 400 mCi (14.8 GBq) 131I-MIBG as compared to a lower dose of 131I-MIBG (4.7 years vs. 1.9 years) [11].

10.2 Further Developments to MIBG Therapy

As commonly available, 131I-MIBG is prepared from stable 127I-MIBG by iodine exchange process. This results in a high proportion of nonradioactive 127I-MIBG in the radiopharmaceutical which competes with the active 131I-MIBG for uptake in the tumor cells, thereby reducing efficacy. Additionally, the high proportion of MIBG can produce sympathomimetic effects. A newer method, the ultratrace method, is available which produces 131I-MIBG of much higher specific activity and is considered carrier free (no carrier added, nca) [12]. Due to the lack of competitive inhibition from 127I-MIBG, the nca 131I-MIBG produces higher concentration in target tissues with similar uptake in nontarget tissues [13].

A new radiopharmaceutical, 211At-meta-astatobenzylguanidine (MABG), is being researched into [14, 15]. 211At is an alpha emitter with a range in tissue of less than 80 μm making it highly cytotoxic. Additionally, the efficacy of alpha particles being independent of tumor growth rate and hypoxia makes them attractive. The short range of the alpha particles reduces the effective range of irradiation, but the irradiated cells can produce toxins which can kill neighboring cells (bystander effect), thus compensating the drawback of limited range of alpha particles [16].

With the development of PRRT agents that bind to the somatostatin receptor, treatment of GEP-NETs with 131I-MIBG has become therapy of second choice.

10.3 Peptide Receptor Radionuclide Therapy

10.3.1 Early Trials with 111In-DTPA-Octreotide

111Indium-diethylenetriaminepentaacetic acid (DTPA)-octreotide (OctreoScan®) was approved by the US Food and Drug Administration in 1994 as an imaging agent. Octreotide binds to the type 2 somatostatin receptors (sst2) which are frequently overexpressed in GEP-NETs and have been successfully used to image sst2-positive tumors. Disintegration of 111-indium produces gamma rays which are used for imaging. The additional emission of Auger and conversion electrons (beta particles) with particle range of a few microns during disintegration led investigators to use 111In-DTPA-octreotide as a PRRT agent.

Early work demonstrated good symptom relief in patients with metastatic neuroendocrine tumors. Anthony et al., on treating patients with at least 2 monthly administrations of 6.7 GBq 111In-DTPA-octreotide, reported symptomatic relief in 62 % of patients, decreased hormonal markers in 81 %, and a partial radiographic response in 8 %. However, partial remission (PR) defined by decrease in size of all lesions by more than 50 % was noted in none of the 26 patients [17]. Valkema et al. observed partial response in one of their 40 patients treated with 20–160 GBq 111In-DTPA-octreotide [18]. The lack of size response in the tumors was not surprising given the relatively small particle range of the emitted particles. Interestingly, Valkema et al. did not observe renal toxicities in any of their patients, one of them having received doses as high as 113 GBq (3.1 Ci). This was surprising as a dose of 100 GBq (2.7 Ci) was expected to deliver 45 Gy to the kidneys—or twice the generally accepted renotoxic dose for external beam radiation. This was taken by the authors to suggest that the short-range Auger electrons originating from urine in the nephrons were not harmful to broader renal function.

10.3.2 90Y-DOTATOC

The next generation of trials used 90Y as the radionuclide. 90Y decays by beta emission averaging 935 keV with a tissue range of 4.0–11.3 mm [2], thereby allowing a greater volume of tissue to be treated. Additionally, a modified somatostatin analog [Tyr^3]octreotide (TOC) with greater affinity to the ss2 receptor was used. The chelating agent was also changed from DTPA to dodecanetetraacetic acid (DOTA). The resulting pharmaceutical 90Y-DOTATOC (Onalta®) thereby had a greater affinity to the ss2 receptor with the 90Y remaining attached for a longer duration of time and irradiating a greater tissue volume.

As can be expected, significantly better results were achieved using 90Y-DOTATOC. Waldherr et al., using 200 mCi (7.4 GBq) administered intravenously in four doses spaced six weeks apart, noted a complete response in 5 % and partial response in 18 % of their 39 patients. Symptomatic relief of diarrhea was noted in 83 % of patients [19]. Similarly, Bushnell et al. reported a favorable clinical outcome in 14 out of their 21 patients after a total of 360 mCi 90Y-DOTATOC (13.2 GBq) in three divided doses at 6–9-week interval [20].

10.3.3 177Lu-DOTATOC/177Lu-DOTATATE

177Lutetium has the advantage of being a gamma as well as a beta emitter, and therefore its in vivo distribution can be imaged. The beta emission from 177Lu averages 47 keV with a tissue range of 0.04–1.8 mm [2]. Replacing the C-terminal threoninol of [Tyr^3]octreotide (TOC) with threonine produces [Tyr^3]octreotate (TATE) and when bound to 177Lu through DOTA produces 177Lu-DOTATATE.

The DOTATATE molecule has been reported to have significantly greater affinity for the sst2 receptors in tumors but no greater uptake in the normal liver, spleen, or kidneys [21].

177Lu-DOTATATE has been recommended as the radiopharmaceutical of choice for PRRT of GEP-NETs [22]. Combination strategies using 90Y to target large tumor masses and 177Lu to target diffuse spread of microscopic disease might be of strategic advantage [23]. Longer survival has been reported by some authors using the dual isotope approach [24]. Patients have reported a quality of life improvement after 177Lu-DOTATATE therapy [25, 26].

10.3.4 Toxicities

In a large series of over 500 patients with GEP-NETs treated with cumulative doses of 750–800 mCi (27.8–29.6 GBq) 177Lu-DOTATATE, Kwekkeboom et al. observed a grade 3 or 4 hematologic toxicity in 3.6 % of patients. In the same study of 310 patients that were followed, 2 % had complete remission, 28 % had partial remission, and 16 % had less than partial response with a 40–72-month survival benefit as compared to historical controls [27].

The long-term effects of 177Lu-DOTATATE on endocrine function have been investigated by Teunissen et al., who observed transient inhibitory effects on spermatogenesis in males and significant decrease of gonadotropins in postmenopausal women. A few patients developed hypothyroidism and elevated HbA_{1c} levels. The authors concluded that 177Lu-DOTATATE was safe in regard to the endocrine system [28].

Octreotide and its derivatives are reabsorbed by the proximal convoluted tubules leading to significant radiation exposure to the kidneys. The kidneys are the rate-limiting organs to PRRT as the 90Y-DOTATOC and 177Lu-DOTATATE are excreted by the kidneys. Renal function loss may manifest years after PRRT, and a decline of creatinine clearance of 7.3 % per year has been reported after 90Y-DOTATOC therapy and 3.8 % per year after 177Lu-DOTATATE therapy [29]. Radiation exposure and consequent radiation damage to the kidneys can be reduced by simultaneous administration of lysine and arginine along with 177Lu-DOTATATE which decreases renal uptake of the radiopharmaceutical [30].

10.3.5 Radiosensitizers

The use of radiosensitizers such as 5-fluorouracil (5-FU) along with PRRT is safe and produces better symptomatic response [22]. Usage of the prodrug of 5-FU, capecitabine, has also been reported and appears to be safe [31]. Increased control on tumor growth has also been reported when capecitabine is used [32].

10.3.6 Locoregional Administration

It is possible to deliver higher tumoricidal doses of radiation to hepatic metastases while minimizing systemic toxicity by delivery of 131I-MIBG or PRRT via the hepatic artery [33, 34]. While current studies demonstrate the safety of locoregional therapy, the incremental value of locoregional therapy over intravenous therapy is difficult to establish.

10.3.7 Other PRRTs

Other pharmaceuticals have also been researched into for PRRT that target receptors different from the sst2. These include peptides that target the gastrin-releasing peptide receptor (GRPR) with potential for imaging and therapy of prostate cancer [35, 36], CCK2 receptors for medullary thyroid cancers and small cell lung cancers [37, 38], and epidermal growth factor targeting gastric, breast, and non-small cell lung cancers [39, 40].

References

1. Krenning EP, Bakker WH, Breeman WA, et al. Localisation of endocrine-related tumours with radioiodinated analogue of somatostatin. Lancet. 1989;1(8632):242–4.
2. Kassis AI, Adelstein SJ. Radiobiologic principles in radionuclide therapy. J Nucl Med. 2005;46 Suppl 1:4S–12.
3. Grunwald F, Ezziddin S. 131I-metaiodobenzylguanidine therapy of neuroblastoma and other neuroendocrine tumors. Semin Nucl Med. 2010;40(2):153–63.
4. Bomanji JB, Papathanasiou ND. (1)(1)(1)In-DTPA(0)-octreotide (Octreoscan), (1)(3)(1)I-MIBG and other agents for radionuclide therapy of NETs. Eur J Nucl Med Mol Imaging. 2012;39 Suppl 1:S113–25.
5. Bomanji J, Levison DA, Flatman WD, et al. Uptake of iodine-123 MIBG by pheochromocytomas, paragangliomas, and neuroblastomas: a histopathological comparison. J Nucl Med. 1987;28(6):973–8.
6. Solanki KK, Bomanji J, Moyes J, Mather SJ, Trainer PJ, Britton KE. A pharmacological guide to medicines which interfere with the biodistribution of radiolabelled meta-iodobenzylguanidine (MIBG). Nucl Med Commun. 1992;13(7):513–21.
7. Giammarile F, Chiti A, Lassmann M, Brans B, Flux G. EANM procedure guidelines for 131I-meta-iodobenzylguanidine (131I-mIBG) therapy. Eur J Nucl Med Mol Imaging. 2008;35(5):1039–47.
8. Castellani MR, Seghezzi S, Chiesa C, et al. (131)I-MIBG treatment of pheochromocytoma: low versus intermediate activity regimens of therapy. Q J Nucl Med Mol Imaging. 2010;54(1):100–13.
9. Mukherjee JJ, Kaltsas GA, Islam N, et al. Treatment of metastatic carcinoid tumours, phaeochromocytoma, paraganglioma and medullary carcinoma of the thyroid with (131)I-meta-iodobenzylguanidine [(131)I-mIBG]. Clin Endocrinol (Oxf). 2001;55(1):47–60.
10. Navalkissoor S, Alhashimi DM, Quigley AM, Caplin ME, Buscombe JR. Efficacy of using a standard activity of (131)I-MIBG therapy in patients with disseminated neuroendocrine tumours. Eur J Nucl Med Mol Imaging. 2010;37(5):904–12.

11. Safford SD, Coleman RE, Gockerman JP, et al. Iodine-131 metaiodobenzylguanidine treatment for metastatic carcinoid. Results in 98 patients. Cancer. 2004;101(9):1987–93.
12. Barrett JA, Joyal JL, Hillier SM, et al. Comparison of high-specific-activity ultratrace 123/131I-MIBG and carrier-added 123/131I-MIBG on efficacy, pharmacokinetics, and tissue distribution. Cancer Biother Radiopharm. 2010;25(3):299–308.
13. Mairs RJ, Boyd M. Optimizing MIBG therapy of neuroendocrine tumors: preclinical evidence of dose maximization and synergy. Nucl Med Biol. 2008;35 Suppl 1:S9–20.
14. Strickland DK, Vaidyanathan G, Friedman HS, Zalutsky MR. Meta-[131I]iodobenzylguanidine uptake and meta-[211At]astatobenzylguanidine treatment in human medulloblastoma cell lines. J Neurooncol. 1995;25(1):9–17.
15. Vaidyanathan G, Strickland DK, Zalutsky MR. Meta-[211At]astatobenzylguanidine: further evaluation of a potential therapeutic agent. Int J Cancer. 1994;57(6):908–13.
16. Mothersill C, Seymour CB. Radiation-induced bystander effects–implications for cancer. Nat Rev Cancer. 2004;4(2):158–64.
17. Anthony LB, Woltering EA, Espenan GD, Cronin MD, Maloney TJ, McCarthy KE. Indium-111-pentetreotide prolongs survival in gastroenteropancreatic malignancies. Semin Nucl Med. 2002;32(2):123–32.
18. Valkema R, De Jong M, Bakker WH, et al. Phase I study of peptide receptor radionuclide therapy with [In-DTPA]octreotide: the Rotterdam experience. Semin Nucl Med. 2002; 32(2):110–22.
19. Waldherr C, Pless M, Maecke HR, et al. Tumor response and clinical benefit in neuroendocrine tumors after 7.4 GBq (90)Y-DOTATOC. J Nucl Med. 2002;43(5):610–6.
20. Bushnell D, O'Dorisio T, Menda Y, et al. Evaluating the clinical effectiveness of 90Y-SMT 487 in patients with neuroendocrine tumors. J Nucl Med. 2003;44(10):1556–60.
21. Kwekkeboom DJ, Bakker WH, Kooij PP, et al. [177Lu-DOTAOTyr3]octreotate: comparison with [111In-DTPAo]octreotide in patients. Eur J Nucl Med. 2001;28(9):1319–25.
22. Kwekkeboom DJ, de Herder WW, van Eijck CH, et al. Peptide receptor radionuclide therapy in patients with gastroenteropancreatic neuroendocrine tumors. Semin Nucl Med. 2010;40(2):78–88.
23. De Jong M, Valkema R, Jamar F, et al. Somatostatin receptor-targeted radionuclide therapy of tumors: preclinical and clinical findings. Semin Nucl Med. 2002;32(2):133–40.
24. Kunikowska J, Krolicki L, Hubalewska-Dydejczyk A, Mikolajczak R, Sowa-Staszczak A, Pawlak D. Clinical results of radionuclide therapy of neuroendocrine tumours with 90Y-DOTATATE and tandem 90Y/177Lu-DOTATATE: which is a better therapy option? Eur J Nucl Med Mol Imaging. 2011;38(10):1788–97.
25. Teunissen JJ, Kwekkeboom DJ, Krenning EP. Quality of life in patients with gastroenteropancreatic tumors treated with [177Lu-DOTA0, Tyr3]octreotate. J Clin Oncol. 2004;22(13): 2724–9.
26. Khan S, Krenning EP, van Essen M, Kam BL, Teunissen JJ, Kwekkeboom DJ. Quality of life in 265 patients with gastroenteropancreatic or bronchial neuroendocrine tumors treated with [177Lu-DOTA0, Tyr3]octreotate. J Nucl Med. 2011;52(9):1361–8.
27. Kwekkeboom DJ, de Herder WW, Kam BL, et al. Treatment with the radiolabeled somatostatin analog [177 Lu-DOTA 0, Tyr3]octreotate: toxicity, efficacy, and survival. J Clin Oncol. 2008;26(13):2124–30.
28. Teunissen JJ, Krenning EP, de Jong FH, et al. Effects of therapy with [177Lu-DOTA 0, Tyr 3] octreotate on endocrine function. Eur J Nucl Med Mol Imaging. 2009;36(11):1758–66.
29. Valkema R, Pauwels SA, Kvols LK, et al. Long-term follow-up of renal function after peptide receptor radiation therapy with (90)Y-DOTA(0), Tyr(3)-octreotide and (177)Lu-DOTA(0), Tyr(3)-octreotate. J Nucl Med. 2005;46 Suppl 1:83S–91.
30. Pool SE, Krenning EP, Koning GA, et al. Preclinical and clinical studies of peptide receptor radionuclide therapy. Semin Nucl Med. 2010;40(3):209–18.
31. van Essen M, Krenning EP, Kam BL, de Herder WW, van Aken MO, Kwekkeboom DJ. Report on short-term side effects of treatments with 177Lu-octreotate in combination with capecitabine in seven patients with gastroenteropancreatic neuroendocrine tumours. Eur J Nucl Med Mol Imaging. 2008;35(4):743–8.

32. Rich TA, Shepard RC, Mosley ST. Four decades of continuing innovation with fluorouracil: current and future approaches to fluorouracil chemoradiation therapy. J Clin Oncol. 2004; 22(11):2214–32.
33. Brogsitter C, Pinkert J, Bredow J, Kittner T, Kotzerke J. Enhanced tumor uptake in neuroendocrine tumors after intraarterial application of 131I-MIBG. J Nucl Med. 2005;46(12):2112–6.
34. McStay MK, Maudgil D, Williams M, et al. Large-volume liver metastases from neuroendocrine tumors: hepatic intraarterial 90Y-DOTA-lanreotide as effective palliative therapy. Radiology. 2005;237(2):718–26.
35. Schroeder RP, van Weerden WM, Bangma C, Krenning EP, de Jong M. Peptide receptor imaging of prostate cancer with radiolabelled bombesin analogues. Methods. 2009;48(2):200–4.
36. Maddalena ME, Fox J, Chen J, et al. 177Lu-AMBA biodistribution, radiotherapeutic efficacy, imaging, and autoradiography in prostate cancer models with low GRP-R expression. J Nucl Med. 2009;50(12):2017–24.
37. Kwekkeboom DJ, Bakker WH, Kooij PP, et al. Cholecystokinin receptor imaging using an octapeptide DTPA-CCK analogue in patients with medullary thyroid carcinoma. Eur J Nucl Med. 2000;27(9):1312–7.
38. Behr TM, Behe M, Angerstein C, et al. Cholecystokinin-B/gastrin receptor binding peptides: preclinical development and evaluation of their diagnostic and therapeutic potential. Clin Cancer Res. 1999;5(10 Suppl):3124s–38.
39. Chen P, Cameron R, Wang J, Vallis KA, Reilly RM. Antitumor effects and normal tissue toxicity of 111In-labeled epidermal growth factor administered to athymic mice bearing epidermal growth factor receptor-positive human breast cancer xenografts. J Nucl Med. 2003;44(9): 1469–78.
40. Cuartero-Plaza A, Martinez-Miralles E, Rosell R, Vadell-Nadal C, Farre M, Real FX. Radiolocalization of squamous lung carcinoma with 131I-labeled epidermal growth factor. Clin Cancer Res. 1996;2(1):13–20.

Chapter 11
Nuclear Medicine Approaches to Treatment of Neuroendocrine Tumors

Ken Herrmann, Rudolf A. Werner, Christina Blümel, and Martin S. Allen-Auerbach

11.1 Nuclear Medicine Approaches for Diagnosis, Staging, Restaging, and Treatment Monitoring of Pancreatic Neuroendocrine Tumors

Neuroendocrine tumors (NETs) often overexpress somatostatin receptors (SSTRs) on the tumor cell surface which may serve as target for diagnosis and treatment; five different somatostatin receptor subtypes have been described: SSTR1, SSTR2, SSTR3, SSTR4, and SSTR5 [1]. Different peptide ligands are available for diagnostic imaging allowing for an in vivo quantification of the SSTR expression and selection of patients potentially benefitting from peptide receptor radionuclide therapy (PRRT) [2].

11.1.1 Somatostatin Receptor Scintigraphy

Until recently ^{111}In-DTPA-octreotide which preferably binds to SSTR2 was most commonly used for diagnostic imaging of NETs [3]. Planar whole-body scans and single photon computed emission tomography (SPECT) are performed 24 h after injection of the radiopharmaceutical [4]. A review including 35 centers reported an overall sensitivity of 85 % (range 57–93 %) and a detection rate of 89 % (67–100 %) by analyzing gastro-entero-pancreatic (GEP)-NETs (grade 1/2) [5]. More recently,

K. Herrmann • R.A. Werner • C. Blümel
Department of Nuclear Medicine, Universitätsklinikum Würzburg, Oberdürrbacher Str. 6, Würzburg 97080, Germany
e-mail: Herrmann_K1@ukw.de; Werner_R1@ukw.de; Bluemel_C@ukw.de

M.S. Allen-Auerbach (✉)
Department of Molecular and Medical Pharmacology, UCLA Medical Center, Medical Plaza 200, Suite B114-61, Los Angeles, CA 90095, USA
e-mail: mauerbach@mednet.ucla.edu

J.R. Pisegna (ed.), *Management of Pancreatic Neuroendocrine Tumors*,
DOI 10.1007/978-1-4939-1798-3_11

introduction of hybrid SPECT/CT scanners provided anatomical correlation. However, small lesions (0.5–1.5 cm) can be missed by the limited resolution of the single photon computed emission tomography/computed tomography (SPECT/CT) technology [4].

11.1.2 Positron Emission Tomography/Computed Tomography (PET/CT)

In Europe, introduction of ^{68}Ga-labeled somatostatin analogs reduced the importance of SPECT tracers. The following three PET tracers are currently used in daily clinical practice: ^{68}Ga-DOTATOC, ^{68}Ga-DOTANOC, and ^{68}Ga-DOTATATE. All three PET tracers show a high affinity for SSTR2. Diagnostic accuracy of ^{68}Ga-DOTATOC and ^{68}Ga-DOTATATE appears to be similar, whereas the wider receptor binding profile of ^{68}Ga-DOTANOC (SSTR2, SSTR3, and SSTR5) compared to ^{68}Ga-DOTATATE (SSTR2) might lead to a better sensitivity [4, 6, 7]. Sensitivity and specificity for detection of NETs were 81 and 90 % for ^{68}Ga-DOTATATE PET/CT [8], identifying significantly more lesions than ^{111}In-DTPA-octreotide [9]. Moreover, PET has a better resolution and the image acquisition of 30–60 min after injection is more patient friendly [4].

^{18}FDG (^{18}F-fluorodeoxy-D-glucose)-PET/CT detects glucose metabolism of tumor cells and should be applied in grade 3 NETs with high proliferation (Ki-67) index: a cutoff value of Ki67 >15 % is associated with a sensitivity of 92 %. In less aggressive cases (grade 1/2) with lower glucose consumption, the detection rate decreases [10].

In order to assess therapy response, treatment monitoring of patients undergoing PRRT should be performed, e.g., functional imaging such as ^{68}Ga-DOTATATE PET/CT but also CT and MRI after 3 months [11].

In summary, NETs can be diagnosed by different peptide ligands allowing for staging, restaging, and selection of patients potentially responding to PRRT. Whereas ^{111}In-DTPA-octreotide has been widely used with a good overall sensitivity for more than a decade, the recent introduction of ^{68}Ga-labeled PET probes has reduced the importance of ^{111}In-DTPA-octreotide because of the inferior image resolution of SPECT imaging. ^{68}Ga-labeled peptide ligands have a higher detection rate of NETs compared to conventional receptor scintigraphy and multi-slice CT [12]. However, in aggressive NETs with high proliferation rates, ^{18}FDG-PET/CT remains the tracer of choice.

11.2 Theranostic Concept of ^{68}Ga and ^{90}Y/^{177}Lu Pairs, Rationale for Therapy

11.2.1 "Theranostic Approach" of NETs

The "theranostic approach" includes tumor diagnosis and tumor treatment using the same peptide ligand labeled with either diagnostic (^{68}Ga/111In) or therapeutic (^{90}Y/177Lu) radioisotopes. Diagnostic imaging allows for staging and restaging, as well as assessment of tumor burden and quantification of target expression for selecting patients who most likely benefit from PRRT. Adequate target expression in tumor tissue is defined as tracer uptake in the tumor above physiologic tracer uptake in the normal liver [13]. NET-relevant therapeutic compounds all have a similar structure: a somatostatin analog is linked to a therapeutic radioisotope by a chelator complex. Showing high affinity towards SSTR2 receptors, these radiolabeled peptide ligands bind to the SSTR2 receptors and are then internalized into the cell and cause apoptosis [14].

In general, PRRT is recommended in inoperable, metastasized cases expressing adequate SSTR on the tumor cell surface [15].

11.2.2 The First Treatment Approaches by Using ^{111}Indium-Octreotide

In the previous decade, Valkema et al. demonstrated longer survival in patients with gastroenteropancreatic tumors undergoing treatment with Auger electron-emitting ^{111}Indium-octreotide [16]. More than half of the patients (21/40) included in this study were noted to have some treatment-induced effect (partial remission, minor remission, or stabilization). In another study, only 2/27 patients (8 %) showed imaging-based morphological partial response (PR) [17]. However, due to the limited tissue penetration, this approach is no longer recommended [13].

Currently, the most commonly used therapeutic radiolabeled somatostatin analogs are ß-emitting ^{90}Y- DOTA-D-Phe-Tyr3-octreotide (DOTATOC) or ß- and y-emitting ^{177}Lu- DOTA-D-Phe-Tyr3-octreotate (DOTATATE):

11.2.3 ^{90}Y-DOTATOC

Waldherr et al. administered 7.4 GBq of ^{90}Y-DOTATOC (4 treatment cycles, time interval of 6 weeks) demonstrating an objective response rate of 38 % in pancreatic NETs [18]. The kidney is one of the most critical organs in patients undergoing treatment with ^{90}Y with a reported treatment-associated decline in creatinine clearance of 7.3 % per year [19].

11.2.4 ^{177}Lu-DOTATATE

In comparison to ^{90}Y-DOTATOC, ^{177}Lu-DOTATATE shows even better response rates: Kwekkeboom and colleagues treated 310 patients with 27.8–29.6 GBq (4 treatment cycles, time interval of 6–10 weeks). The median OS was 46 months with CR in 2 % and PR in 28 % of patients, respectively [20]. Focusing on PNETs, a German research group analyzed a patient cohort of 68 end-stage pancreatic NETs

(PNETs) (grade 1/2) and were able to demonstrate a PR in 60 % with a median OS of 53 months. As expected, a G1 status was associated with a significantly ($p=0.044$) longer PFS and OS [21]. Thus, ^{177}Lu-DOTATATE seems to be a highly effective treatment option in advanced PNETs. Patients with advanced NETs showing initial response to PRRT but suffering from progressive disease during long-term follow-up were retreated and analyzed retrospectively: CR was found in 3 % and PR in 18 % of patients, respectively, and none of those patients showed severe side effects. Thus, a retreatment approach as "salvage therapy" is not only feasible but also effective [22].

11.2.5 Combination of ^{90}Y-DOTATOC and ^{177}Lu-DOTATATE

There are several studies analyzing the effect of combining both radiolabeled compounds: Villard et al. compared a single injection of ^{90}Y-DOTATOC versus a combination of ^{90}Y-DOTATOC and ^{177}Lu-DOTATATE suggesting some advantages for the combination procedure (OS, 5.51 years (combination) vs. 3.96 years (alone)) [23]. However, to our knowledge this approach has not gained wide acceptance for routine use.

11.2.6 Indications and Contraindications

According to *The joint IAEA, EANM, and SNMMI practical guidance on peptide receptor radionuclide therapy in neuroendocrine tumours*, the indications for PRRT are the following:

- Positive histopathology
- Positive SSTR2 expression on tumor surface confirmed by OctreoScan© or ^{68}Ga-DOTATOC PET/CT
- Metastatic or inoperable NET
- NET grade 1 or 2 according to the WHO 2010 classification
- Ki-67</=20 %
- Karnofsky performance status >60 % or EGOC performance <2 [11]

Absolute and relative contraindications:

- Pregnancy, breastfeeding
- Renal impairment (creatinine clearance <40–50 mL/min)
- Impaired hematological function (Hb <5 mmol/L (8 g/dL), platelets $<75\times10^9$/L, WBC$<2\times10^9$/L)
- Severe hepatic impairment: total bilirubin >3 × upper limit of normal or albumin <30 g/L and prothrombin time increased
- Severe cardiac impairment [13]

11.3 Procedure of PRRT: Patient Preparation, Administration, and Acute/Delayed Side Effects

11.3.1 Pretherapeutic Procedure: Patient Preparation

In order to avoid saturation of SSTR, somatostatin analogs should be discontinued: the last injection of long-acting analogs should occur 4–6 weeks prior to PRRT and short-acting compounds can be given up to 1 day before treatment [11].

PRRT should be performed according to local legislation and the multidisciplinary tumor board. The nuclear medicine department should provide trained staff including physicians, radiochemists, and medical physicist. Radiation safety arrangements are required.

Due to the potential nephrotoxicity of PRRT, pretherapeutic assessment of renal function is mandatory: a venous blood sample, 24 h urine collection, and/or renal scintigraphy should be performed prior to PRRT, e.g., Tc-99m mercaptoacetyltriglycine (MAG3) and Tc-99m diethylene triamine penta-acetic acid (DTPA) scintigraphy especially in patients with a clinical suspicion for impaired renal function [2].

11.3.2 Administration

Under physician observation the radiopharmaceutical diluted in 10–100 mL normal saline should be infused over 10–30 min through a peripheral intravenous line. The infusion system should be flushed with saline after completion of the administration (9).

Since the coadministration of amino acids (AA) significantly reduces nephrotoxicity by limiting renal absorption of the radiopeptide, it has been implemented into guidelines. Different renal protection protocols exist, but the most frequently applied algorithm is the so-called single-day 50 g protection protocol: on the day of therapy, 2,000 mL of normal saline solution containing 25 g of arginine hydrochloride and 25 g of lysine hydrochloride is administered over 4 h (starting 30 min to 1 h prior to PRRT and continuing for a total of 3–3.5 h after therapy, with the infusion pump set to 250 mL/h) [2, 11]. The infusion of positively charged AA usually causes a transient hyperkalemia: a Swiss research group reported on hyperkalemia (>5.0 mmol/L) in more than ¾ of patients undergoing treatment with PRRT. Blood values reached their maximum 4 h after AA infusion with the highest potassium level measured as 6.7 mmol/L [24]. In most of the patients, therapy-induced hyperkalemia resolved after 24 h, but in critical cases (symptomatic with palpitations, malaise, ECG changes indicating hyperkalemia), immediate treatment is required (e.g., intravenous infusion of insulin and glucose) [24, 25].

11.3.3 Acute and Delayed Side Effects

Analyzing 479 patients undergoing PRRT with more than 1,500 treatment cycles, hormonal release-induced crisis occurs only in 1 % (up to 48 h after administration). Within 24 h, 9 % of patients suffered from abdominal pain and 35 % complained of nausea and vomiting [20, 26]. For the latter, serotonin 5-HT3 receptor antagonist can be given prophylactically, e.g., ondansetron 8 mg [20].

Delayed side effects mostly consist of serious renal impairment and myelosuppression [20, 21]. The acceptable maximum absorbed dose for the bone marrow is 2 Gy [27]: Bodei et al. reported that a cumulative dose of 29 GBq ^{177}Lu-DOTATATE (7.4 GBq/treatment cycle) was well tolerated and led to a cumulative bone marrow dose of <1.5 Gy [28]. Thus, 3–5 treatment cycles with a time interval of 6–12 weeks per cycle of administering ^{177}Lu-DOTATATE/^{177}Lu-DOTATOC are feasible. Reversible alopecia has also been described as a delayed side effect in 62 % of patients (10).

A complete blood cell count, as well as renal and liver function tests, is recommended every 12 weeks for the first year after PRRT. In case of clinical risk factors, these examinations should be repeated at least twice in the following year [11].

11.4 Outlook Including High Dose, Radiosensitization, Combination with Chemotherapy, Transcatheter Arterial Chemoembolization (TACE), and Selective Internal Radiation Therapy (SIRT)

11.4.1 Combination with Radiosensitizing and Chemotherapeutic Drugs

In order to make tumor cells more sensitive to PRRT, radiosensitizing chemotherapeutic drugs such as capecitabine have been given to patients receiving four treatment cycles with standard activity of ^{177}Lu-octreotate: almost all patients of this cohort showed PR and/or SD of 94 % [29]. Claringbold et al. administered ^{177}Lu-octreotate in combination with capecitabine and temozolomide in advanced low-grade NETs demonstrating 90 % survival at 2-year follow-up [30].

11.4.2 Locoregional Procedures in Case of Discontinuing PRRT

NETs are known to metastasize to the liver: if PRRT has to be discontinued because of side effects or tumor progression, locoregional therapy might be helpful.

Ezzidin et al. reported a median OS of 29 months for a patient cohort with liver-dominant metastasis receiving injection of ^{90}Yttrium microspheres into

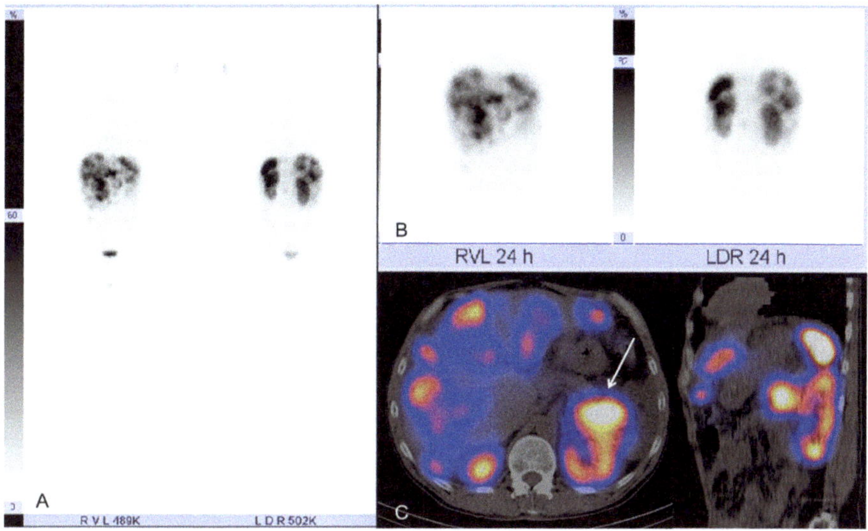

Fig. 11.1 ^{111}In-DTPA-octreotide scan of a 55-year-old male suffering from pancreatic NET with liver metastasis. (**a**) Whole-body scan (anterior and posterior view) showing SSTR-positive liver metastases. (**b**) Extract of whole-body scan showing abdominal region. (**c**) SPECT/CT showing pancreatic NET (*white arrow*) with liver metastases

the liver (SIRT [31]). TACE and TAE (transarterial embolization) are commonly performed in order to induce necrosis by obstructing the afferent vessel: both are effective in advanced NETs. TAE appears to be associated with fewer occurrences of post-embolization syndrome including fever, pain, nausea, and vomiting [32] (Fig. 11.1).

11.4.3 Outlook: Role of Dosimetry, "High-Dose" Approach in PRRT, Neoadjuvant Treatment

Dosimetry has the potential of minimizing treatment-induced kidney and bone marrow damage. Currently, a dose of up to 7.4 GBq is considered to be safe as administered activity per cycle [33]. Forrer et al. reported high interpatient variability of bone marrow absorbed doses. By calculating the effective dose to the rate-limiting target organs (kidneys and bone marrow), it would be theoretically possible to calculate patient-specific treatment doses of ^{177}Lu-DOTATATE in order to avoid under- or overtreatment, minimize side effects, and be able to administer the maximum activity per treatment cycle [34].

Neoadjuvant treatment with PRRT prior to surgery presents another potential application of PRRT, although this has not been studied sufficiently to date [35, 36] (Fig. 11.2).

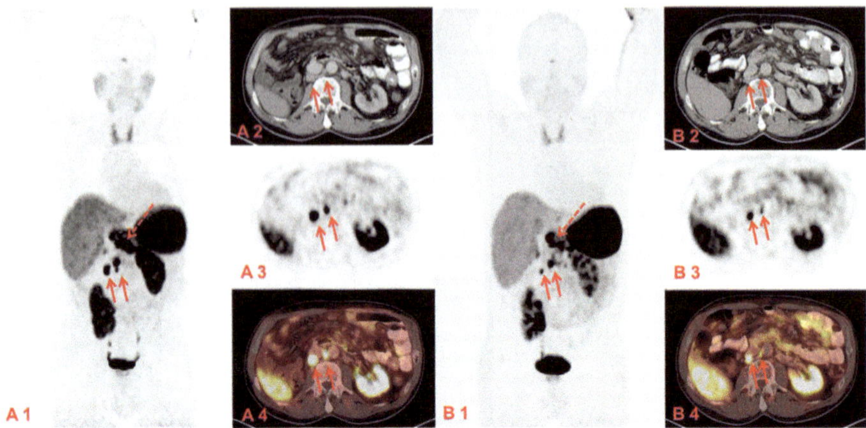

Fig. 11.2 Pretherapeutic (**A1–4**) and post-therapeutic (**B1–4**) ^{68}Ga-DOTATOC PET/CT scans of a 62-year-old male with a pancreatic NET and abdominal lymph node metastases undergoing two cycles of PRRT with a cumulative dose of 15.6 GBq ^{177}Lu-DOTATATE indicating size reduction of abdominal lymph nodes (partial response). Pretherapeutic (**A1**) and post-therapeutic (**B1**) MIPs (anterior view) displaying the pancreatic neuroendocrine primary tumor (*dotted arrow*) and the abdominal lymph node metastases (*solid arrows*). Corresponding pretherapeutic (**A2–4**) and post-therapeutic (**B2–4**) trans-axial CT (**A2, B2**), PET (**A3, B3**), and fused PET/CT (**A4, B4**) displaying the abdominal lymph nodes (*solid arrows*)

11.5 Summary

NETs normally overexpress somatostatin receptors on the tumor cell surface which can be used as a target for nuclear medicine diagnosis and treatment of NETs. In a "theranostic approach," assessment of tumor burden using SSTR-PET/CT as a functional imaging modality is helpful in selecting patients for treatment with PRRT. The accuracy of ^{68}Ga-labeled somatostatin analogs for staging of NETs exceeds that of conventional receptor scintigraphy (octreotide SPECT) and anatomical imaging modalities such as CT and MRI.

PRRT is recommended for patient with inoperable and metastasized NETs expressing SSTR. The most commonly administered therapeutic radiopeptides are ^{90}Yttrium-DOTATOC and ^{177}Lu-DOTATATE. PRRT is generally considered a well-tolerated and a safe therapy: acute side effects are nausea and vomiting but also life-threatening hyperkalemia.

References

1. Modlin IM, Oberg K, Chung DC, Jensen RT, de Herder WW, Thakker RV, et al. Gastroenteropancreatic neuroendocrine tumours. Lancet Oncol. 2008;9(1):61–72.
2. Virgolini I, Ambrosini V, Bomanji JB, Baum RP, Fanti S, Gabriel M, et al. Procedure guidelines for PET/CT tumour imaging with 68Ga-DOTA-conjugated peptides: 68Ga-DOTA-TOC,

68Ga-DOTA-NOC, 68Ga-DOTA-TATE. Eur J Nucl Med Mol Imaging. 2010; 37(10):2004–10.
3. de Herder WW, Hofland LJ, van der Lely AJ, Lamberts SW. Somatostatin receptors in gastroentero-pancreatic neuroendocrine tumours. Endocr Relat Cancer. 2003;10(4):451–8.
4. Sundin A. Radiological and nuclear medicine imaging of gastroenteropancreatic neuroendocrine tumours. Best Pract Res Clin Gastroenterol. 2012;26(6):803–18.
5. Modlin IM, Kidd M, Latich I, Zikusoka MN, Shapiro MD. Current status of gastrointestinal carcinoids. Gastroenterology. 2005;128(6):1717–51.
6. Wild D, Bomanji JB, Benkert P, Maecke H, Ell PJ, Reubi JC, et al. Comparison of 68Ga-DOTANOC and 68Ga-DOTATATE PET/CT within patients with gastroenteropancreatic neuroendocrine tumors. J Nucl Med. 2013;54(3):364–72.
7. Poeppel TD, Binse I, Petersenn S, Lahner H, Schott M, Antoch G, et al. 68Ga-DOTATOC versus 68Ga-DOTATATE PET/CT in functional imaging of neuroendocrine tumors. J Nucl Med. 2011;52(12):1864–70.
8. Haug AR, Cindea-Drimus R, Auernhammer CJ, Reincke M, Wangler B, Uebleis C, et al. The role of 68Ga-DOTATATE PET/CT in suspected neuroendocrine tumors. J Nucl Med. 2012;53(11):1686–92.
9. Srirajaskanthan R, Kayani I, Quigley AM, Soh J, Caplin ME, Bomanji J. The role of 68Ga-DOTATATE PET in patients with neuroendocrine tumors and negative or equivocal findings on 111In-DTPA-octreotide scintigraphy. J Nucl Med. 2010;51(6):875–82.
10. Binderup T, Knigge U, Loft A, Mortensen J, Pfeifer A, Federspiel B, et al. Functional imaging of neuroendocrine tumors: a head-to-head comparison of somatostatin receptor scintigraphy, 123I-MIBG scintigraphy, and 18F-FDG PET. J Nucl Med. 2010;51(5):704–12.
11. Bodei L, Mueller-Brand J, Baum RP, Pavel ME, Horsch D, O'Dorisio MS, et al. The joint IAEA, EANM, and SNMMI practical guidance on peptide receptor radionuclide therapy (PRRNT) in neuroendocrine tumours. Eur J Nucl Med Mol Imaging. 2013;40(5):800–16.
12. Gabriel M, Decristoforo C, Kendler D, Dobrozemsky G, Heute D, Uprimny C, et al. 68Ga-DOTA-Tyr3-octreotide PET in neuroendocrine tumors: comparison with somatostatin receptor scintigraphy and CT. J Nucl Med. 2007;48(4):508–18.
13. Kwekkeboom DJ, Krenning EP, Lebtahi R, Komminoth P, Kos-Kudla B, de Herder WW, et al. ENETS consensus guidelines for the standards of care in neuroendocrine tumors: peptide receptor radionuclide therapy with radiolabeled somatostatin analogs. Neuroendocrinology. 2009;90(2):220–6.
14. Waser B, Tamma ML, Cescato R, Maecke HR, Reubi JC. Highly efficient in vivo agonist-induced internalization of sst2 receptors in somatostatin target tissues. J Nucl Med. 2009;50(6):936–41.
15. Auernhammer CJ, Goke B. Therapeutic strategies for advanced neuroendocrine carcinomas of jejunum/ileum and pancreatic origin. Gut. 2011;60(7):1009–21.
16. Valkema R, De Jong M, Bakker WH, Breeman WA, Kooij PP, Lugtenburg PJ, et al. Phase I study of peptide receptor radionuclide therapy with [In-DTPA]octreotide: the Rotterdam experience. Semin Nucl Med. 2002;32(2):110–22.
17. Anthony LB, Woltering EA, Espenan GD, Cronin MD, Maloney TJ, McCarthy KE. Indium-111-pentetreotide prolongs survival in gastroenteropancreatic malignancies. Semin Nucl Med. 2002;32(2):123–32.
18. Waldherr C, Pless M, Maecke HR, Schumacher T, Crazzolara A, Nitzsche EU, et al. Tumor response and clinical benefit in neuroendocrine tumors after 7.4 GBq (90)Y-DOTATOC. J Nucl Med. 2002;43(5):610–6.
19. Valkema R, Pauwels SA, Kvols LK, Kwekkeboom DJ, Jamar F, de Jong M, et al. Long-term follow-up of renal function after peptide receptor radiation therapy with (90)Y-DOTA(0), Tyr(3)-octreotide and (177)Lu-DOTA(0), Tyr(3)-octreotate. J Nucl Med. 2005;46 Suppl 1:83S–91.
20. Kwekkeboom DJ, de Herder WW, Kam BL, van Eijck CH, van Essen M, Kooij PP, et al. Treatment with the radiolabeled somatostatin analog [177 Lu-DOTA 0, Tyr3]octreotate: toxicity, efficacy, and survival. J Clin Oncol. 2008;26(13):2124–30.

21. Ezziddin S, Khalaf F, Vanezi M, Haslerud T, Mayer K, Al Zreiqat A, et al. Outcome of peptide receptor radionuclide therapy with 177Lu-octreotate in advanced grade 1/2 pancreatic neuro-endocrine tumours. Eur J Nucl Med Mol Imaging. 2014;41(5):925–33.
22. Sabet A, Haslerud T, Pape UF, Ahmadzadehfar H, Grunwald F, Guhlke S, et al. Outcome and toxicity of salvage therapy with 177Lu-octreotate in patients with metastatic gastroenteropan-creatic neuroendocrine tumours. Eur J Nucl Med Mol Imaging. 2014;41(2):205–10.
23. Villard L, Romer A, Marincek N, Brunner P, Koller MT, Schindler C, et al. Cohort study of somatostatin-based radiopeptide therapy with [(90)Y-DOTA]-TOC versus [(90)Y-DOTA]-TOC plus [(177)Lu-DOTA]-TOC in neuroendocrine cancers. J Clin Oncol. 2012; 30(10):1100–6.
24. Giovacchini G, Nicolas G, Freidank H, Mindt TL, Forrer F. Effect of amino acid infusion on potassium serum levels in neuroendocrine tumour patients treated with targeted radiopeptide therapy. Eur J Nucl Med Mol Imaging. 2011;38(9):1675–82.
25. Weisberg LS. Management of severe hyperkalemia. Crit Care Med. 2008;36(12):3246–51.
26. de Keizer B, van Aken MO, Feelders RA, de Herder WW, Kam BL, van Essen M, et al. Hormonal crises following receptor radionuclide therapy with the radiolabeled somatostatin analogue [177Lu-DOTA0, Tyr3]octreotate. Eur J Nucl Med Mol Imaging. 2008;35(4): 749–55.
27. Nonstochastic effects of ionizing radiation ICRP Publication 41. Ann. ICRP 14 (3), 1984. http://www.icrp.org/publication.asp?id=ICRP%20Publication%2041.
28. Bodei L, Cremonesi M, Grana CM, Fazio N, Iodice S, Baio SM, et al. Peptide receptor radio-nuclide therapy with (1)(7)(7)Lu-DOTATATE: the IEO phase I-II study. Eur J Nucl Med Mol Imaging. 2011;38(12):2125–35.
29. Claringbold PG, Brayshaw PA, Price RA, Turner JH. Phase II study of radiopeptide 177Lu-octreotate and capecitabine therapy of progressive disseminated neuroendocrine tumours. Eur J Nucl Med Mol Imaging. 2011;38(2):302–11.
30. Claringbold PG, Price RA, Turner JH. Phase I-II study of radiopeptide 177Lu-octreotate in combination with capecitabine and temozolomide in advanced low-grade neuroendocrine tumors. Cancer Biother Radiopharm. 2012;27(9):561–9.
31. Ezziddin S, Meyer C, Kahancova S, Haslerud T, Willinek W, Wilhelm K, et al. 90Y Radioembolization after radiation exposure from peptide receptor radionuclide therapy. J Nucl Med. 2012;53(11):1663–9.
32. Fiore F, Del Prete M, Franco R, Marotta V, Ramundo V, Marciello F, et al. Transarterial embo-lization (TAE) is equally effective and slightly safer than transarterial chemoembolization (TACE) to manage liver metastases in neuroendocrine tumors. Endocrine. 2014.
33. Krenning EP, Kwekkeboom DJ, Bakker WH, Breeman WA, Kooij PP, Oei HY, et al. Somatostatin receptor scintigraphy with [111In-DTPA-D-Phe1]- and [123I-Tyr3]-octreotide: the Rotterdam experience with more than 1000 patients. Eur J Nucl Med. 1993;20(8):716–31.
34. Forrer F, Krenning EP, Kooij PP, Bernard BF, Konijnenberg M, Bakker WH, et al. Bone marrow dosimetry in peptide receptor radionuclide therapy with [177Lu-DOTA(0), Tyr(3)]octreotate. Eur J Nucl Med Mol Imaging. 2009;36(7):1138–46.
35. Sowa-Staszczak A, Pach D, Chrzan R, Trofimiuk M, Stefańska A, Tomaszuk M, Kołodziej M, et al. Peptide receptor radionuclide therapy as a potential tool for neoadjuvant therapy in patients with inoperable neuroendocrine tumours (NETs). Eur J Nucl Med Mol Imaging. 2011;38(9):1669–74.
36. Barber TW, Hofman MS, Thomson BN, Hicks RJ. The potential for induction peptide receptor chemoradionuclide therapy to render inoperable pancreatic and duodenal neuroendocrine tumours resectable. Eur J Surg Oncol. 2012;38(1):64–71.

Chapter 12
Novel Targets for Future Medical Treatments

Sandy T. Liu, Andrew E. Hendifar, and Edward M. Wolin

12.1 Introduction

Pancreatic neuroendocrine tumors (pNETs) are heterogeneous in morphological, functional, and clinical features. Although they are generally slow growing and indolent, the incidence and prevalence of pNETs are rising. 64 % of patients present with distant metastases and have a median survival time of only 24 months [1]. In contrast to poorly differentiated pNETs, well-differentiated pNETs have a relatively limited response to standard chemotherapy. This is due to their low mitotic rate (Ki-67 levels of ≤2), high levels of bcl-2, and expression of genes related to chemoresistance [2, 3]. Fortunately, there have been recent developments in our understanding of the molecular signaling pathways underlying tumor progression in pNETs. The PI3K/AKT/mTOR pathway is one of the most important pathways implicated in the pathogenesis of pNETs as gene expression as this pathway is altered in the majority of pNETs. Furthermore, amplified angiogenesis is a distinguishing feature of well-differentiated pNETs. They are highly vascularized tumors, with increased expression of EGF, PDGF, IGF-1, and VEGF, providing opportunities

S.T. Liu, M.D.
Department of Medicine, Cedars-Sinai Medical Center, 8700 Beverly Blvd., Suite 1042AC, Los Angeles, CA 90048, USA

A.E. Hendifar, M.D., M.P.H.
Department of Gastrointestinal Oncology, Samuel Oschin Cancer Center, Cedars-Sinai Medical Center, 8700 Beverly Blvd., Suite 1042AC, Los Angeles, CA 90048, USA
e-mail: andrew.hendifar@cshs.org

E.M. Wolin, M.D. (✉)
Carcinoid and Neuroendocrine Tumor Program Medical Oncology, Samuel Oschin Cancer Center, Cedars-Sinai Medical Center, 8700 Beverly Blvd., Suite 1042AC, Los Angeles, CA 90048, USA
e-mail: edward.wolin@cshs.org

J.R. Pisegna (ed.), *Management of Pancreatic Neuroendocrine Tumors*,
DOI 10.1007/978-1-4939-1798-3_12

Table 12.1 Angiogenesis Inhibitors

Angiogenesis inhibitors			
Mathew Kulke, 2006	Temozolomide + bevacizumab	Phase II	Completed
Stanford Cancer Center	Capecitabine, temozolomide, and bevacizumab	Phase II	Ongoing
Mathew Kulke, 2007	Everolimus and octreotide ± bevacizumab	Phase II	Ongoing
Multikinase inhibitors			
Eric Raymond, 2011	Sunitinib	Phase III	Completed
Timothy Hobday, 2007	Sorafenib	Phase II	Completed
Jennifer Chan, 2009	Sorafenib + everolimus	Phase I	Ongoing
Alexandra Phan, 2010	Pazopanib + octreotide LAR	Phase II	Completed
Juame Capdevilla, 2011	Pazopanib	Phase II	Ongoing
Halla Nimeiri, 2011	Pazopanib and temozolomide	Phase I/II	Ongoing
mTOR inhibitors			
Jennifer Chan, 2007	Everolimus and temozolomide	Phase I/II	Ongoing
Juan Valle, 2012	BEZ235 vs. everolimus	Phase II	Ongoing
Patrick J. Loehrer, 2012	BEZ235 after failure of mTOR inhibitor therapy	Phase II	Ongoing
James Yao, 2011	Octreotide LAR ± everolimus	Phase III	Completed
James Yao, 2011	Everolimus	Phase III	Completed
Juan Valle, 2011	Everolimus ± pasireotide LAR	Phase II	Ongoing
Insulin growth factor inhibitors			
Mathew Kulke, MD	Ganitumab	Phase II	Completed
Leonard Saltz, MD	Dalotuzumab	Phase II	Completed
James Yao, MD	Cixutumumab, everolimus, and octreotide LAR	Phase I	Ongoing

for therapies targeting angiogenesis. Until recently, there were few therapeutic options for well-differentiated pNETs, and the use of somatostatin analogs had become the mainstay of therapy in terms of symptomatic relief and tumor stabilization. New targeted biological agents with everolimus and sunitinib are providing new treatment options for the management of advanced pNETs with the potential of other novel agents detailed in this chapter for further improved survival outcomes for patients in the coming years (Table 12.1).

12.2 PI3K/AKT/mTOR Pathway

The recent success of everolimus, an inhibitor of the mammalian target of rapamycin, is a proof of principle that the phosphatidylinositol 3-kinase (PI3K)/Akt/mammalian target of rapamycin (mTOR) pathway is important to pNET tumorigenesis and progression [1, 2]. There are substantial preclinical findings over the past two decades that need to be reviewed in light of this significant clinical success. Furthering our understanding of this vital pathway will lead to enhanced therapies for patients with pNET.

mTOR is an intracellular serine–threonine kinase and a component of the phosphatidylinositol 3′ kinase (PI3K)/AKT signaling pathway. It comprises mTOR complex-1 (mTORC1) and mTOR complex-2 (mTORC2), which regulate cellular function including proliferation, survival, and angiogenesis. mTORC1 is composed of mTOR, regulatory-associated protein of mTOR (Raptor), and target of rapamycin complex subunit LST8. mTORC1 regulates cellular transcription and translation via downstream MTORC1 substrates. These are eukaryotic translation initiation factor 4E-binding protein-1 (4EBP-1) and ribosomal S6 kinase-1 (S6K1). S6K1 inhibits the PI3K/AKT pathway and is part of a negative feedback loop on PI3K/AKT signaling. mTORC2 consists of mTOR and target of rapamycin complex subunit LST8, rapamycin-insensitive companion of mTOR (rictor), and mitogen-activated protein kinase-associated protein-1. The role of mTORC2 is less well defined, but is known to directly phosphorylate Akt in the PI3K/Akt pathway.

Multiple endocrine neoplasia type I (MEN1), tuberous sclerosis complex (TSC), neurofibromatosis type I, and von Hippel–Lindau (VHL) disease are genetic disorders associated with an increased incidence of pNETS. Across these syndromes, mutations in well-defined oncogenes and tumor suppressor genes lead to constitutive activation of the PI3K/Akt/mTOR pathway. Recently, alterations in PI3K/Akt/mTOR pathway have been implicated in sporadic pNETS tumorigenesis justifying its exploitation as a target for rationale therapy [3–5].

The PI3K/AKT/mTOR pathway plays an important role in cellular proliferation, growth, and metabolism. The phosphoinositide 3-kinase (PI3K) family of lipid kinases phosphorylate the 3'-hydroxyl group of phosphoinositides and are composed of three classes (I–III) with distinct lipid products, substrate specificity, and functionality [6]. Class I PI3Ks are divided into two subfamilies (classes 1A and 1B), depending on the receptors to which they couple. Class IA PI3Ks are the most widely implicated class in human cancers and are activated by receptor tyrosine kinases [7]. Once activated, PI3K catalyzes conversion plasma membrane lipidphosphatidylinositol-4,5-bisphosphate [PI(4,5)P2] (PIP2) to phosphatidylinositol-3,4,5-trisphosphate [PI(3,4,5)P3] (PIP3) [8]. The end result of PI3K activation is the generation of PIP3 and downstream activation of AKT and other proteins [9].

PIP3 is tightly regulated by PIP3 phosphatases (PTEN, SHIP1, and SHIP2) which return PIP3 to PIP2 [10]. The most important to cancer propagation is phosphatase and tensin homolog (PTEN) [11]. Although PTEN has activity against multiple substrates [12], its PIP3 phosphatase activity has been implicated as its tumor suppressor function through studies of the inherited cancer syndromes (Cowden's specifically) [11].

PIP3 helps to activate AKT, a serine–threonine kinase also known as protein kinase B. The AKT family consists of three highly conserved members: AKT1, AKT2, and AKT3. AKT1 is the isoform most studied in cancers, AKT2 is found in tissues responding to insulin, and AKT3 is found in the brain [13]. When PI3K is activated, all three isoforms of AKT are translocated from the cytoplasm to the plasma membrane and are phosphorylated by phosphoinositide-dependent kinase 1

Table 12.2 Incidence of PI3K/Akt/mTOR pathway alterations in pNET

Pathway alteration	Incidence	Tumor type	Reference
mTOR overexpression	6/9 (67 %)	Poorly differentiated pNET	Shida et al. [24]
Mutations in *PTEN*, *TSC2*, *PIK3CA*	10/68 (15 %)	pNET	Jiao et al. [19]
Akt activation	28/46 (61 %)	NET	Ghayouri et al. [28]
TSC2 and PTEN protein alterations	61/72 (85 %)	Primary pNETs	Missiaglia et al. [18]

PI3K phosphatidylinositol 3-kinase, *pNET* pancreatic neuroendocrine tumor, *PTEN* phosphatase and tensin homolog, *mTOR* mammalian target of rapamycin, *TSC2* tuberous sclerosis protein 2

(PDK1) and potential PDK2, thereby transforming all AKT isoforms to their active form [10, 14, 15]. Active AKT further phosphorylates and activates several downstream effectors.

Akt is a key regulator of PI3K and mTOR signaling and therefore is an important driver of malignant progression and chemoresistance. Activated Akt can phosphorylate the tumor suppressor protein, tuberous sclerosis protein 2 (TSC2 or tuberin), to attenuate its negative regulation of the PI3K pathway through mTOR inhibition [13]. The biological effects of AKT include the regulation of cell survival, proliferation, and angiogenesis through regulation of insulin growth factor, nuclear factor Kb, p53, cyclin D1, mTOR, and HIF-1α [10].

12.3 Relevance of PI3K/AKT/mTOR Pathway to pNET

Tumor sequencing data, immunohistochemical expression, and gene expression profiling of neuroendocrine tumors have implicated the PI3K/Akt/mTOR pathway in pNET tumorigenesis (see Table 12.2.) The majority of pNETs overexpress mTOR [16] and many harbor mutations and alterations in PTEN, TSC2, and PIK3CA [3, 4]. Expression profiling in pNETs demonstrates marked alteration in genes associated with this pathway [3, 17]. Akt activation is prevalent and associated with poor differentiation [16, 18].

Activation of this pathway is likely driven by dysregulated tyrosine kinases and enhanced signaling by vascular endothelial and insulin growth factors. Studies demonstrate that druggable tyrosine kinase receptors including PDGFR, EGFR, and c-kit are overexpressed in endocrine pancreatic tumors [19, 20]. NETs and NET cell lines frequently express both IGFs and the IGF-1R receptor suggesting autocrine and/or paracrine signaling [21, 22]. IGF-1R binding leads to the direct activation of signaling cascades in the MAPK and P13k kinase pathways [23]. The clinical benefit from somatostatin analogs in insulin growth factor secreting tumors suggests an important interplay in pNET tumorigenesis [24].

Antiangiogenic therapeutic approaches are also promising as pNETs are highly vascular with increased expression of vascular endothelial growth factor [25] and its associated receptor [26]. Activation of the PI3K pathway may also be led by the overexpression of VEGFR1 in the companion vasculature suggesting an interaction between this pathway and angiogenesis [2]. Mutations in the *FLT1/VEGFR1* gene have been detected in pNET cell lines [2].

Investigations of the PI3K/AKT/mTOR pathway in pNETs reveal an association between its activation and cancer development. Both TSC2 and phosphatase and tensin homolog (PTEN) are key negative regulators of the PI3K/Akt/mTOR pathway [27] and were found to be suppressed in a large panel of 72 primary pNET tumor samples (including matched metastases) that were analyzed by tissue microarray gene expression analysis [3]. The low expression of TSC2 and PTEN was significantly associated with more aggressive tumors and shorter disease-free and overall survival [3]. MicroRNA expression profiling shows that the genetic regulator miR-21 [28, 29] and nuclear proliferation marker protein Ki-67 index are inversely proportional to PTEN levels [3, 28]. The overexpression of miR-21 is strongly associated with both a high Ki-67 proliferation index and the presence of liver metastasis [29].

AKT regulation appears to be important to pNET tumorigenesis. Activation of Akt has been reported in 28/46 (61 %) NET tumor samples, and 76 % of all NETs display constitutive AKT phosphorylation. *MEN1* gene mutations, the hallmark of MEN syndromes, have been found in 27/100 (27 %) clinically sporadic pNETs, including 23/75 (30 %) nonfunctioning pNETs and 4/25 (16 %) functioning pNETs [2, 30]. Menin loss has also been associated with Akt activation in a mouse model of pancreatic islet adenoma [31].

The downstream effector of the PI3K-activated signaling pathway is mTOR, and its expression in NETs is associated with metastasis and proliferation. mTOR is overexpressed in well-differentiated pNETs [32]. In one study, mTOR overexpression was also seen in poorly differentiated pNETs 6/9 (67 %), which comprise the more aggressive forms of the tumor [18].

12.4 Success Targeting the PI3K/Akt/mTOR Pathway

Everolimus (RAD001, 40-O-(2 hydroxyethyl) derivative of rapamycin), an oral rapamycin analog, selectively inhibits mTORC1. As a result of in vitro activity of rapamycin and its associated analogs [33–35], the RADIANT-1 (RAD001 in advanced neuroendocrine tumors 1) study was designed to study the use of everolimus in patients with neuroendocrine tumors [36]. RADIANT-1 was a phase II trial in patients with pNET refractory to chemotherapy and stratified according to octreotide therapy. 160 patients with progressive islet cell carcinoma were assigned to either everolimus 10 mg daily alone or everolimus 10 mg daily plus octreotide LAR. The overall response rate (ORR) by central radiological review was 9.6 % for everolimus alone and 4.4 % for the combined use, with stable disease (SD) rates of 67.8 % and 80.0 %, respectively. The median progression-free survival (PFS) was 9.7 months for everolimus alone and 16.7 months everolimus and octreotide LAR.

These promising results in a cancer that was historically chemotherapy resistant led to the RADIANT-2 study [37]. 429 patients with advanced low- to intermediate-grade carcinoid tumors and a history of hormone-related symptoms were enrolled into RADIANT-2. All patients received octreotide LAR and were otherwise randomized to everolimus 10 mg daily vs. placebo. PFS by central review was 16.4 months in the everolimus-plus-octreotide LAR group and 11.3 months in the placebo-plus-octreotide LAR group.

In order to validate these results in a large prospective study, RADIANT-3 was initiated [1]. This landmark study was the largest phase III pNET trial to date. 410 patients with advanced, low-grade, or intermediate-grade pNET to were randomized to everolimus 10 mg/day or placebo. Everolimus was superior to placebo in prolonging progression-free survival from 11 months vs. 4.6 months, a 65 % reduction in estimated risk of progression or death. Similar benefit in disease stability was seen in those enrolled in the everolimus arm (73 vs. 51 % for everolimus and placebo). Overall response rates were low, but higher in the everolimus arm (5 vs. 2 %, $p+0.001$). Benefit was irrespective of age, gender, race, performance status, prior treatment, or tumor grade.

Single-agent everolimus clearly demonstrates clinical benefit in the treatment of pNETS despite its low objective response rate. Everolimus is active against mTORC1 only, and low response rates may reflect the drug's inability to prevent mTORC2-mediated activation of Akt [38]. New treatments targeting both mTORC 1 and mTORC 2 are in development and may improve efficacy. In addition, combination therapy targeting upstream (PI3K inhibitors) or downstream (Akt) to the mTORC complexes may prevent PI3K/Akt/mTOR pathway activation and reactivation. As such, recent investigations and ongoing studies have focused on inhibitors of alternate components of the PI3K/Akt/mTOR pathway, dual target inhibitors, and effective combination chemotherapies.

12.5 Potential Targets in the PI3K/Akt/mTOR Pathway

The PI3K/Akt/mTOR pathway is complex, and perturbations can occur at multiple sites. Therefore, there are several potential targets and combinations of therapies compelling for further investigation. The rapamycin analogs (rapalogs), specifically everolimus, are the most clinically advanced and the furthest developed class of inhibitors. These agents inhibit the complex mTORC1. Two well-characterized mTORC1 substrates are eukaryotic translation initiation factor 4E-binding protein-1 and ribosomal S6 kinase-1 (S6K1), both regulating transcription and translation initiation of critical growth genes. However, S6K1 is part of a negative feedback loop on PI3K/Akt signaling via suppression of the insulin receptor substrate-1 (IRS1), which links IGF-1 to the PI3K pathway. mTORC2 is less defined than mTORC1, but is known to mediate Akt phosphorylation on serine-473, which is required for full Akt activity in the PIK3/Akt/mTOR signaling cascade. A potential limitation of inhibiting mTORC1 therefore arises as a result of the S6K1/IRS1 negative feedback loop that can leave mTORC2 capable of perpetuating Akt activity [39].

Inhibitors of Akt either compete with ATP at the active site or bind distally to the catalytic site, inducing a conformational change that prevents ligand binding. Akt inhibition may be expected to abrogate negative feedback loops perpetuated by mTORC2 following mTORC1 inhibition [39]. Agents that inhibit both mTOR complexes may also overcome this problem. Therefore, inhibitors of both mTORC1 and mTORC2 and AKT inhibitors are attractive drug candidates.

Potential PI3K/Akt/mTOR pathway targets upstream of mTOR are the PI3K proteins themselves. Three classes (I–III) of PI3K have been characterized that vary in structure and substrate preference. The class I enzymes are activated directly by cell-surface receptors, and it is the catalytic domain of the class IA PI3K p110 subunits that are the most widely implicated in cancer [40]. Pan-PI3K inhibitors target all four class I p110 isoforms; however, PI3K inhibitors specific for individual class I p110 isoforms may allow for anticancer activity with an improved safety profile. The majority of therapeutic interventions or drugs under investigation are pan-p110 inhibitors, although a number of PI3K-targeted agents with isoform specificity have now been reported [38, 41]. It is of potential clinical significance that dual inhibition of PI3K and mTORC1/2 may be mediated through the shared structural homology between the catalytic domains of the PI3K p110 subunits and mTORC1/2 [7]. Agents that target both PI3K and mTOR will likely lead to improved inhibition of this pathway.

12.6 Novel PI3K/AKT/mTOR Inhibitors

12.6.1 Chaperone Heat Shock Protein 90 Inhibitors

Preclinical data are suggesting unique PI3K/Akt/mTOR pathway inhibitors in pNET. This can be achieved either through direct inhibition of specific pathway proteins or through indirect inhibition of molecular chaperones. The molecular chaperone heat shock protein 90 (HSP90) is overexpressed in a number of tumors and is an emerging target for anticancer therapy. The potential activity of the HSP90 inhibitor IPI-504 has been studied in pNET cells, and this agent inhibited the growth of human insulinoma and pancreatic carcinoid cells by approximately 70 % [42]. IPI-504 downregulated IGF-1 and a number of proteins in the PI3K/Akt/mTOR pathway. Combination of IPI-504 with mTOR or Akt inhibitors also led to additive effects and is a promising combination.

12.6.2 PI3K Inhibitors

Although the regulation of VEGF synthesis and secretion in pNET cells is complex, the involvement of the PI3K/mTOR/hypoxia-inducible factor (HIF)-1/VEGF pathway in the angiogenesis of predominantly hypervascular pNETs has prompted the study of upstream pathway inhibition with PI3K and mTOR inhibitors [43].

A combination of the PI3K inhibitor (LY294002) and an mTOR inhibitor (rapamycin) decreased VEGF secretion by murine endocrine cell lines STC-1, INS-r3, and INS-r9. Intracellular levels of HIF-1α were decreased concomitantly with VEGF levels, suggesting inhibition of the PI3K/Akt/mTOR/HIF-1/VEGF pathway [43].

12.6.3 AKT Inhibitors

Akt inhibition has been explored and validated in a number of preclinical studies. Triciribine, a direct Akt inhibitor, reduced the growth of pNET cells (by either triciribine monotherapy or combination therapies) [42]. Insulinoma (CM) or gut NET cells (STC-1) treated with triciribine significantly reduced tumor cell growth by 59 % and 65 %, respectively. In contrast, triciribine did not inhibit the BON pancreatic tumor cell line, which overexpress PTEN [42]. The pan-Akt inhibitor perifosine inhibits both Akt phosphorylation and cell viability in human pancreatic BON1 and other NET cells. Perifosine was shown to suppress the phosphorylation of downstream targets, including MDM2 and p70S6K, to suppress NET cell viability and colony-forming capacity [44]. Studies on individual Akt isoforms using siRNA transfection also suggest a prominent role for Akt1 and Akt3 in NET signaling and highlight the potential for selective Akt targeting in pNET.

A number of small-molecule Akt inhibitors with varying potencies and specificities for Akt isoforms have been developed. Adenosine triphosphate (ATP)-competitive Akt inhibitors are promiscuous and have a higher likelihood of off-target effects. Allosteric Akt inhibitors are more specific and have been preferred for clinical studies in patients with pNET. Results from a phase I trial of MK-2206, an oral non-ATP-competitive allosteric inhibitor of Akt, have now been reported [45]. In 33 patients with solid tumors, two patients with advanced pNET had minor responses, achieving tumor shrinkages of −13.1 % and −17.5 %, respectively. The latter of these two patients experienced marked reduction in ascites and peripheral edema, and tumor central necrosis. Akt blockade was confirmed in this study by an observed reduction in phosphorylated serine-473 Akt in all tumor biopsies assessed [45]. Reversible hyperglycemia and increases in insulin c-peptide also confirmed target response. Drug-related toxicities included skin rash (52 %), nausea (36 %), and pruritus (24 %). Combination trials have been initiated with MK-2206 with either standard chemotherapy (carboplatin, paclitaxel, docetaxel) or targeted agents (including lapatinib [human epidermal growth factor receptor 2/EGFR inhibitor], ridaforolimus [mTORC1 inhibitor], and AZD6244 [MEK1/2 inhibitor]).

12.6.4 Protein Kinase C (PKC) Inhibitors

In addition to its role in PI3K-mediated cell signaling, Akt is a downstream target of serine–threonine protein kinase C (PKC). The PKC family members play central regulatory roles in cell cycle progression, differentiation, tumorigenesis, apoptosis, and secretion [46, 47]. Dysregulation of PKC signaling is implicated in tumor development and progression [48]. Enzastaurin, an oral serine–threonine kinase inhibitor, has been developed as a PKCβ-selective inhibitor. Preclinical data suggests that it suppresses PKC signaling, inhibits angiogenesis, and abrogating the PI3K/Akt/mTOR pathway [49]. It reduces the phosphorylation of Akt and the proliferation of BON1 pNET cells [50]. These preclinical data suggest a promising future for this agent in the treatment of pNETs.

12.6.5 Combination PI3K/AKT/mTOR Pathway Inhibitors

Multi-target inhibition of the PI3K/AKT/mTOR pathway will hopefully overcome the treatment resistance and feedback mechanisms characteristic of mTORC1 inhibition. The dual mTORC1/mTORC2 inhibitor CC-223 has recently been selected for clinical evaluation based on its potential ability to address mTORC2-mediated escape mechanisms and resistance. In an ongoing phase I/II study in patients with solid and hematologic malignancies, a cohort of patients with NETs was included [51]. Evidence of preliminary antitumor activity has been demonstrated, including one durable partial response, although to date only gastrointestinal NETs of non-pancreatic origin have been investigated.

Dual inhibition of mTOR and upstream targets has been a focus of recent investigations. The dual PI3K/mTOR inhibitor NVP-BEZ235 has proved to be a more efficient inducer of apoptosis and cell cycle arrest than single inhibitors in various NET cell lines. NVP-BEZ235 prevented both vertical and horizontal negative feedback activation of Akt after treatment with everolimus [52]. This appears in the clinic to be a promising approach [53]. The combination of everolimus, NVP-BEZ235, and the RAF inhibitor RAF265 was also more effective than treatment with a single kinase inhibitor. RAF265 inhibits ERK1/2 phosphorylation and strongly induces Akt phosphorylation and VEGF secretion (possibly due to Akt-mediated HIF-1α activation), suggesting a further compensatory feedback loop on PI3K/Akt signaling in pNETs [52]. The IGF-1R inhibitor NVP-AEW541has demonstrated dual targeting inhibition of the downstream PI3K/Akt/mTOR and RAS/RAF/MEK pathways [54]. These data provide a strong rationale for combination therapies directed at PI3K/Akt/mTOR signaling and RAS/RAF/MEK signaling in pNETs. A number of inhibitors of the PI3K/Akt/mTOR pathway are currently being evaluated in pNETs or NETs, both alone and in combination regimens.

12.7 Tyrosine Kinase Inhibitors

Sunitinib (Sutent®, SU11248, Pfizer) is an oral inhibitor of the receptor tyrosine kinases of VEGFR-1 and VEGFR-2, PDGFR-α and PDGFR-β, c-KIT, and FMS-like tyrosine kinase-3 (FLT3) [55]. Sunitinib has been shown in numerous preclinical studies to reduce tumor proliferation [56]. Antitumor activity in pNET was demonstrated in a phase II study [57] enrolling 12 Japanese patients with unresectable, well-differentiated tumors. Each patient received 37.5 mg daily of sunitinib, and the clinical benefit rate was 75 %, the objective response rate was 50 %, and 11/12 observed some tumor shrinkage after 1 month of initiation of treatment. Impressively, progression-free survival (PFS) was 91 % at 6 months and 71 % at 12 months [57]. In another phase II study, among pNET patients treated with sunitinib 50 mg daily, the overall objective response rate (ORR) was 16.7 %, 6-month stable disease rate 68.2 %, and 1-year survival rate 81.1 %. The median time to tumor progression was 7.7 months. Patient-reported outcome data also showed no significant differences from baseline quality of life or fatigue during treatment [58].

Sutent has also been used in conjunction with local therapies. In a study by Strosberg et al., sunitinib was shown to delay tumor revascularization and extend PFS following hepatic artery embolization for advanced pNET. Serum VEGF levels increased by 34 % ($p=0.03$) following arterial embolization. The overall response rate was 72 %, and median PFS was 15.2 months. Survival of 95 % (95 % CI, 0.88–1.00) at 1 year and 59 % at 5 years (95 % CI, 0.38–0.80) was encouraging. This supports a possible role of sunitinib, a VEGFR inhibitor, following embolization therapy [59].

In the subsequent phase III study [60] that ultimately led to the approval of sunitinib in 2011 for treatment of patients with advanced, well-differentiated pNET in both Europe and the United States, sunitinib was shown to have a dramatic advantage over placebo. In this trial, 171 patients with progressive metastatic pNET were randomized to receive either placebo or sunitinib 37.5 mg daily. Patients were allowed to crossover to sunitinib at the time of tumor progression and give patients randomized to placebo access to open-label sunitinib. Early study termination occurred since the primary endpoint was met, and there were more severe adverse events and deaths in the placebo arm. As a result, the early discontinuation of the study precluded definitive hypothesis looking for differences in PFS between sunitinib and placebo. Nevertheless, progression-free survival was doubled in sunitinib-treated patients compared with placebo (11.4 vs. 5.5 months for placebo, $p<0.001$) and an increase in the response rate (9 vs. 0 %, $p=0.007$). There was no survival benefit with sunitinib on further follow-up with a median OS of 33 months in the sunitinib group vs. 26.7 months in the placebo group ($p=0.115$) likely due to treatment crossover obscuring the endpoint [61]. Subgroup analysis revealed sunitinib had a PFS advantage regardless of prior treatment with somatostatin analogs or chemotherapy, Ki-67 expression, and extent of tumor burden. Despite the crossover, there was still an improvement in survival in patients treated with sunitinib that seemed to be maintained over time. These results were in agreement with the radiological response rate.

There were no major differences in quality of life and level of fatigue between the sunitinib and placebo groups, although adverse events were more common in the sunitinib group. The most frequent side effects of sunitinib included neutropenia, hypertension, hand–foot syndrome, abdominal pain, diarrhea, and fatigue [60]. Sunitinib has become a standard of care in patients with unresectable, advanced, metastatic pNET.

12.8 Angiogenesis (VEGF) Inhibitors

Angiogenesis plays a fundamental role in tumor growth and development. Most well-differentiated pNETs are high vascularized expressing high levels of VEGF. VEGF is a potent promoter of endothelial cell activation for new tumor vessel formation and appears to be the most important growth factor regulating physiologic and pathologic angiogenesis [62]. It is also a key driver in metastatic spread since early revascularization occurs during tumor formation [63]. The concept of angiogenesis-dependent tumor growth and the targeted blocking of blood flow to the tumor for cancer treatment was initially established by Folkman in the early 1970s [64]. Among the VEGF receptor family, VEGFR-1 and VEGFR-2, when bound to VEGF, are the main regulator of angiogenesis and are frequently overexpressed in certain solid tumors, including NETs, and have been associated with tumor progression [25, 26, 65]. Patients with weak or strong VEGF expression developed metastasis more frequently, compared with patients who did not express VEGF, 58 % vs. 14 % ($p=0.03$), respectively. Additionally, in patients with weak VEGF expression, the median PFS was 81 months compared with 29 months in patients with strong VEGF expression ($p=0.02$) [5]. The VEGF/VEGFR system has been extensively studied to be a promising target in the treatment of pNET.

Bevacizumab (Avastin®) is a humanized monoclonal antibody directed against VEGF, preventing binding to its receptors, VEGFR-1 and VEGFR-2. It is currently indicated for treating several types of tumors including metastatic colorectal cancer, nonsquamous non-small cell lung cancer, glioblastoma multiforme, and metastatic renal cell carcinoma [66]. Bevacizumab has been investigated either alone or in combination with other drugs in NET with promising results. In a phase II study, patients with advanced carcinoid tumors were randomly assigned to treatment with either bevacizumab or IFNα_{2b} added to octreotide LAR for 18 weeks. In the bevacizumab arm, 5 % of patients had disease progression compared with 32 % treated with pegylated IFN$\alpha_{2b.}$ Bevacizumab dramatically decreased tissue perfusion documented by functional CT monitoring. Yao et al. observed a decrease in tumor blood flow among patients treated with bevacizumab at day 2 and week 18 (49 % ($p<0.01$) and 28 % ($p<0.01$), respectively). Four of 22 patients treated with bevacizumab achieved radiographic partial responses. Conversely, there was no significant change in tumor blood flow seen in patients treated with pegylated IFN$_{2b.}$ In the bevacizumab arm, there was almost a 30 % higher rate of PFS after 18 weeks compared to the peg-IFNα_{2b} arm (95 % PFS vs. 68 % PFS). The reported survival rates were 93 %, 67 %, and 56 % for 1, 2, and 3 years, respectively [67]. Based on these positive findings, a phase III study randomizing 400 patients with small bowel carcinoids to receive either bevacizumab or peg-IFN$_{2b}$ in addition to octreotide has completed enrollment (Southwest Oncology Group, SWOG S0518 trial; NCT00569127). This may be a key trial that will define the role of VEGF inhibitors in carcinoids.

Building on the recent trials showing efficacy of mTOR inhibitors alone, a randomized phase II study comparing mTOR inhibitor alone with the combination of mTOR inhibitor and bevacizumab in patients with pNETs may help define the potential additive activity of bevacizumab in pNETs. Chan and colleagues found bevacizumab and temozolomide combination appears to be promising for patients with pNETs as there was a 24 % response rate in pNETs but 0 % in carcinoid tumors [68]. In another recently completed phase II study, the combination of everolimus and bevacizumab was shown to be well tolerated and had a 26 % response rate in patients with advanced NET [69]. Given these results, the National Cancer Institute (NCI) has an ongoing phase II study randomizing patients with locally advanced or metastatic pNETs not amenable to surgery to receive everolimus and octreotide with or without bevacizumab to assess antitumor activity and toxicity of the regimen [CALGB 80701; NCT01229943]. Another phase II study of bevacizumab plus temsirolimus in pNET has been reported (NCT01010126). There are also several current ongoing studies with bevacizumab in combination with chemotherapeutic agents that appears to be promising. In particular, a phase II study of 31 patients, bevacizumab plus capecitabine and oxaliplatin resulted in PR in seven patients (23 %), of which six of seven of these patients had pNET (35).

12.9 IGF/IGFR Inhibitors

IGF-1, IGF-2, and their tyrosine kinase receptor, IGF-1R, are involved in the development and progression of NET and is an autocrine regulator of NET [22]. Targeting IGF/IGF-1R has been suggested as a novel therapy for pNETs as preclinical data has shown that somatostatin analogs and mTOR inhibitors exhibit antitumor activity through the IGF-1 signaling pathway. After activation of IGF-1R by IGF-1 and IGF-2, signals are transmitted via elements of the PI3K/AKT/mTOR and the Ras/Raf/MEK/ERK pathways enhancing cell proliferation and promoting survival in tumor cells [70]. In a study by von Wichert, IGF-1 was shown to be a major autocrine regulator of neuroendocrine secretion and growth of human BON cells (human pancreatic carcinoid-derived endocrine-like cells that express IGF-1R and secrete IGF-1). They were shown to stimulate the release of chromogranin A when exogenously IGF-1 was added. Equally, blocking IGF-1 prompted a marked inhibition of basal chromogranin A secretion [22]. NET has been shown to have increased expression of IGFs. mRNA of both IGF-1 and IGF-1R were found in most of the samples from 54 patients with Zollinger–Ellison syndrome [71]. Furthermore, increased expression of both IGF-1 and IGF-1R was associated with greater tumor burden, growth, and aggressiveness. There was also a correlation with IGF-1R and the incidence of liver metastasis and with disease-free survival [71].

There are currently several studies that use different approaches to block the components of the IGF-1R pathway. MK-0646 is a humanized IgG1 monoclonal antibody that binds to IGF-1. It has been shown to be safe and well tolerated in patients with solid tumors [72]. A phase II study of MK-0646 monotherapy in 25 patients (15 carcinoids, 10 pancreatic NETs) revealed that MK-6046 was inactive as a single agent [73]. Based on this study, MK-0646 does not have sufficient activity for further study as monotherapy and is currently being studied in combination with conventional chemotherapy with advanced pancreatic, breast, and non-small cell lung cancer.

NVP-AEW541 is a novel selective IGF-1R tyrosine kinase inhibitor that has been shown to be active in BON cells and a human insulinoma cell line. The antineoplastic effects of NVP-AEW541 involve the inactivation of ERK1/2. NVP-AEW541 caused apoptosis and cell cycle arrest and inhibited NET cell proliferation in a dose-dependent fashion. Moreover, there was an increase in the antiproliferative properties when NVP-AEW541 was combined with doxorubicin and fluvastatin [74]. AMG 479 (ganitumab) is a humanized monoclonal antibody to IGFR-1, preventing the binding of IGF-1 and IGF-2 to IGF-1R. It has been studied in a phase I trial which showed one patient with pNET had a complete response lasting for 28 months. It also showed one partial response and one minor response in two patients with NETs [75]. Cixutumumab (IMC-A12) is another fully human IgG1 antibody against IGF-1R being studied in patients with NETs. There is an ongoing phase I study with the combination of cixutumumab, everolimus, and octreotide LAR in patients with advanced NETs (NCT01204476).

12.10 Immunotherapy

Several different immunotherapy approaches are currently being studied in targeting cytotoxic T-lymphocyte antigen 4 and PD-1 in NET. Dendritic cells play a central role in initiation and immunization leading to immune memory, making them ideal in presenting tumor material to cytotoxic T cells [76]. One small study conducted by Schott et al. used dendritic cell-based immunotherapy to treat patients with metastatic pNET. The patient's dendritic cells were generated from peripheral blood monocytes and were loaded with tumor-derived lysate which were then delivered by subcutaneous injections in 4-week intervals. Not only did patients develop delayed hypersensitivity skin reaction, with skin biopsy demonstrating a strong perivascular and epidermal infiltration with CD4 and CD8 positive, but the DC-based vaccination was also noted to have a decrease in tumor marker chromogranin A. Tumor regression was also seen on ultrasound [77].

12.11 Summary

For the first time in over 20 years, the survival and outlook for pNET have changed due to a better understanding of the pathogenesis and cell signaling pathways to identify potential new targets. Both sunitinib and everolimus symbolize a new phase in the development of targeted and combination therapy for advanced pNETs. These therapies are effective at improving disease-free survival, even in previously treated patients, and have changed the daily clinical management of patients with progressive advanced pNETs. Furthermore, we have gained new insights to help treat these tumors, and more breakthroughs are coming. This is truly an exciting and optimistic era for patients with pNETs.

References

1. Yao JC, Shah MH, Ito T, Bohas CL, Wolin EM, Van Cutsem E, et al. Everolimus for advanced pancreatic neuroendocrine tumors. N Engl J Med. 2011;364(6):514–23.
2. Corbo V, Beghelli S, Bersani S, Antonello D, Talamini G, Brunelli M, et al. Pancreatic endocrine tumours: mutational and immunohistochemical survey of protein kinases reveals alterations in targetable kinases in cancer cell lines and rare primaries. Ann Oncol. 2012; 23(1):127–34.
3. Missiaglia E, Dalai I, Barbi S, Beghelli S, Falconi M, della Peruta M, et al. Pancreatic endocrine tumors: expression profiling evidences a role for AKT-mTOR pathway. J Clin Oncol. 2010;28(2):245–55.
4. Jiao Y, Shi C, Edil BH, de Wilde RF, Klimstra DS, Maitra A, et al. DAXX/ATRX, MEN1, and mTOR pathway genes are frequently altered in pancreatic neuroendocrine tumors. Science. 2011;331(6021):1199–203.
5. Zhang J, Jia Z, Li Q, Wang L, Rashid A, Zhu Z, et al. Elevated expression of vascular endothelial growth factor correlates with increased angiogenesis and decreased progression-free survival among patients with low-grade neuroendocrine tumors. Cancer. 2007;109(8):1478–86.
6. Cantley LC. The phosphoinositide 3-kinase pathway. Science. 2002;296(5573):1655–7.
7. Engelman JA, Luo J, Cantley LC. The evolution of phosphatidylinositol 3-kinases as regulators of growth and metabolism. Nat Rev Genet. 2006;7(8):606–19.
8. Katso R, Okkenhaug K, Ahmadi K, White S, Timms J, Waterfield MD. Cellular function of phosphoinositide 3-kinases: implications for development, homeostasis, and cancer. Annu Rev Cell Dev Biol. 2001;17:615–75.
9. Inukai K, Funaki M, Ogihara T, Katagiri H, Kanda A, Anai M, et al. p85alpha gene generates three isoforms of regulatory subunit for phosphatidylinositol 3-kinase (PI 3-Kinase), p50alpha, p55alpha, and p85alpha, with different PI 3-kinase activity elevating responses to insulin. J Biol Chem. 1997;272(12):7873–82.
10. Vivanco I, Sawyers CL. The phosphatidylinositol 3-Kinase AKT pathway in human cancer. Nat Rev Cancer. 2002;2(7):489–501.
11. Myers MP, Pass I, Batty IH, Van der Kaay J, Stolarov JP, Hemmings BA, et al. The lipid phosphatase activity of PTEN is critical for its tumor suppressor function. Proc Natl Acad Sci U S A. 1998;95(23):13513–8.
12. Tamura M, Gu J, Matsumoto K, Aota S, Parsons R, Yamada KM. Inhibition of cell migration, spreading, and focal adhesions by tumor suppressor PTEN. Science. 1998;280(5369): 1614–7.
13. Inoki K, Li Y, Zhu T, Wu J, Guan KL. TSC2 is phosphorylated and inhibited by Akt and suppresses mTOR signalling. Nat Cell Biol. 2002;4(9):648–57.
14. Andjelković M, Alessi DR, Meier R, Fernandez A, Lamb NJ, Frech M, et al. Role of translocation in the activation and function of protein kinase B. J Biol Chem. 1997;272(50):31515–24.
15. Bellacosa A, Chan TO, Ahmed NN, Datta K, Malstrom S, Stokoe D, et al. Akt activation by growth factors is a multiple-step process: the role of the PH domain. Oncogene. 1998; 17(3):313–25.
16. Catena L, Bajetta E, Milione M, Ducceschi M, Valente M, Dominoni F, et al. Mammalian target of rapamycin expression in poorly differentiated endocrine carcinoma: clinical and therapeutic future challenges. Target Oncol. 2011;6(2):65–8.
17. Perren A, Komminoth P, Saremaslani P, Matter C, Feurer S, Lees JA, et al. Mutation and expression analyses reveal differential subcellular compartmentalization of PTEN in endocrine pancreatic tumors compared to normal islet cells. Am J Pathol. 2000;157(4):1097–103.

18. Shida T, Kishimoto T, Furuya M, Nikaido T, Koda K, Takano S, et al. Expression of an activated mammalian target of rapamycin (mTOR) in gastroenteropancreatic neuroendocrine tumors. Cancer Chemother Pharmacol. 2010;65(5):889–93.
19. Fjällskog ML, Lejonklou MH, Oberg KE, Eriksson BK, Janson ET. Expression of molecular targets for tyrosine kinase receptor antagonists in malignant endocrine pancreatic tumors. Clin Cancer Res. 2003;9(4):1469–73.
20. Zhang L, Smyrk TC, Oliveira AM, Lohse CM, Zhang S, Johnson MR, et al. KIT is an independent prognostic marker for pancreatic endocrine tumors: a finding derived from analysis of islet cell differentiation markers. Am J Surg Pathol. 2009;33(10):1562–9.
21. Nilsson O, Wängberg B, Theodorsson E, Skottner A, Ahlman H. Presence of IGF-I in human midgut carcinoid tumours–an autocrine regulator of carcinoid tumour growth? Int J Cancer. 1992;51(2):195–203.
22. von Wichert G, Jehle PM, Hoeflich A, Koschnick S, Dralle H, Wolf E, et al. Insulin-like growth factor-I is an autocrine regulator of chromogranin A secretion and growth in human neuroendocrine tumor cells. Cancer Res. 2000;60(16):4573–81.
23. Wang Y, Sun Y. Insulin-like growth factor receptor-1 as an anti-cancer target: blocking transformation and inducing apoptosis. Curr Cancer Drug Targets. 2002;2(3):191–207.
24. Lamberts SW, van der Lely AJ, de Herder WW, Hofland LJ. Octreotide. N Engl J Med. 1996;334(4):246–54.
25. Terris B, Scoazec JY, Rubbia L, Bregeaud L, Pepper MS, Ruszniewski P, et al. Expression of vascular endothelial growth factor in digestive neuroendocrine tumours. Histopathology. 1998;32(2):133–8.
26. Christofori G, Naik P, Hanahan D. Vascular endothelial growth factor and its receptors, flt-1 and flk-1, are expressed in normal pancreatic islets and throughout islet cell tumorigenesis. Mol Endocrinol. 1995;9(12):1760–70.
27. Ghayouri M, Boulware D, Nasir A, Strosberg J, Kvols L, Coppola D. Activation of the serine/theronine protein kinase Akt in enteropancreatic neuroendocrine tumors. Anticancer Res. 2010;30(12):5063–7.
28. Capdevila J, Tabernero J. A shining light in the darkness for the treatment of pancreatic neuroendocrine tumors. Cancer Discov. 2011;1(3):213–21.
29. Roldo C, Missiaglia E, Hagan JP, Falconi M, Capelli P, Bersani S, et al. MicroRNA expression abnormalities in pancreatic endocrine and acinar tumors are associated with distinctive pathologic features and clinical behavior. J Clin Oncol. 2006;24(29):4677–84.
30. Corbo V, Dalai I, Scardoni M, Barbi S, Beghelli S, Bersani S, et al. MEN1 in pancreatic endocrine tumors: analysis of gene and protein status in 169 sporadic neoplasms reveals alterations in the vast majority of cases. Endocr Relat Cancer. 2010;17(3):771–83.
31. Wang Y, Ozawa A, Zaman S, Prasad NB, Chandrasekharappa SC, Agarwal SK, et al. The tumor suppressor protein menin inhibits AKT activation by regulating its cellular localization. Cancer Res. 2011;71(2):371–82.
32. Kasajima A, Pavel M, Darb-Esfahani S, Noske A, Stenzinger A, Sasano H, et al. mTOR expression and activity patterns in gastroenteropancreatic neuroendocrine tumours. Endocr Relat Cancer. 2011;18(1):181–92.
33. Grozinsky-Glasberg S, Franchi G, Teng M, Leontiou CA, Ribeiro de Oliveira A, Dalino P, et al. Octreotide and the mTOR inhibitor RAD001 (everolimus) block proliferation and interact with the Akt-mTOR-p70S6K pathway in a neuro-endocrine tumour cell Line. Neuroendocrinology. 2008;87(3):168–81.
34. Zitzmann K, De Toni EN, Brand S, Göke B, Meinecke J, Spöttl G, et al. The novel mTOR inhibitor RAD001 (everolimus) induces antiproliferative effects in human pancreatic neuroendocrine tumor cells. Neuroendocrinology. 2007;85(1):54–60.
35. Moreno A, Akcakanat A, Munsell MF, Soni A, Yao JC, Meric-Bernstam F. Antitumor activity of rapamycin and octreotide as single agents or in combination in neuroendocrine tumors. Endocr Relat Cancer. 2008;15(1):257–66.
36. Yao JC, Phan AT, Chang DZ, Wolff RA, Hess K, Gupta S, et al. Efficacy of RAD001 (everolimus) and octreotide LAR in advanced low- to intermediate-grade neuroendocrine tumors: results of a phase II study. J Clin Oncol. 2008;26(26):4311–8.

37. Pavel ME, Hainsworth JD, Baudin E, Peeters M, Hörsch D, Winkler RE, et al. Everolimus plus octreotide long-acting repeatable for the treatment of advanced neuroendocrine tumours associated with carcinoid syndrome (RADIANT-2): a randomised, placebo-controlled, phase 3 study. Lancet. 2011;378(9808):2005–12.
38. Markman B, Dienstmann R, Tabernero J. Targeting the PI3K/Akt/mTOR pathway–beyond rapalogs. Oncotarget. 2010;1(7):530–43.
39. O'Reilly KE, Rojo F, She QB, Solit D, Mills GB, Smith D, et al. mTOR inhibition induces upstream receptor tyrosine kinase signaling and activates Akt. Cancer Res. 2006; 66(3):1500–8.
40. Liu P, Cheng H, Roberts TM, Zhao JJ. Targeting the phosphoinositide 3-kinase pathway in cancer. Nat Rev Drug Discov. 2009;8(8):627–44.
41. Knight ZA, Gonzalez B, Feldman ME, Zunder ER, Goldenberg DD, Williams O, et al. A pharmacological map of the PI3-K family defines a role for p110alpha in insulin signaling. Cell. 2006;125(4):733–47.
42. Gloesenkamp CR, Nitzsche B, Ocker M, Di Fazio P, Quint K, Hoffmann B, et al. AKT inhibition by triciribine alone or as combination therapy for growth control of gastroenteropancreatic neuroendocrine tumors. Int J Oncol. 2012;40(3):876–88.
43. Villaume K, Blanc M, Gouysse G, Walter T, Couderc C, Nejjari M, et al. VEGF secretion by neuroendocrine tumor cells is inhibited by octreotide and by inhibitors of the PI3K/AKT/mTOR pathway. Neuroendocrinology. 2010;91(3):268–78.
44. Zitzmann K, Vlotides G, Brand S, Lahm H, Spöttl G, Göke B, et al. Perifosine-mediated Akt inhibition in neuroendocrine tumor cells: role of specific Akt isoforms. Endocr Relat Cancer. 2012;19(3):423–34.
45. Yap TA, Yan L, Patnaik A, Fearen I, Olmos D, Papadopoulos K, et al. First-in-man clinical trial of the oral pan-AKT inhibitor MK-2206 in patients with advanced solid tumors. J Clin Oncol. 2011;29(35):4688–95.
46. Hug H, Sarre TF. Protein kinase C isoenzymes: divergence in signal transduction? Biochem J. 1993;291(Pt 2):329–43.
47. Musashi M, Ota S, Shiroshita N. The role of protein kinase C isoforms in cell proliferation and apoptosis. Int J Hematol. 2000;72(1):12–9.
48. Podar K, Tai YT, Davies FE, Lentzsch S, Sattler M, Hideshima T, et al. Vascular endothelial growth factor triggers signaling cascades mediating multiple myeloma cell growth and migration. Blood. 2001;98(2):428–35.
49. Capurso G, Fazio N, Festa S, Panzuto F, De Braud F, Delle FG. Molecular target therapy for gastroenteropancreatic endocrine tumours: biological rationale and clinical perspectives. Crit Rev Oncol Hematol. 2009;72(2):110–24.
50. Molè D, Gagliano T, Gentilin E, Tagliati F, Pasquali C, Ambrosio MR, et al. Targeting protein kinase C by Enzastaurin restrains proliferation and secretion in human pancreatic endocrine tumors. Endocr Relat Cancer. 2011;18(4):439–50.
51. Shih KC, Bendell J, Reinert, Jones, Kelley, Infante, et al. Phase I trial of an oral TORC1/TORC2 inhibitor (CC-223) in advanced solid and hematologic cancers. American Society of Clinical Oncology; Chicago: J Clin Oncol. 2012.
52. Zitzmann K, Rüden J, Brand S, Göke B, Lichtl J, Spöttl G, et al. Compensatory activation of Akt in response to mTOR and Raf inhibitors: a rationale for dual-targeted therapy approaches in neuroendocrine tumor disease. Cancer Lett. 2010;295(1):100–9.
53. Serra V, Markman B, Scaltriti M, Eichhorn PJ, Valero V, Guzman M, et al. NVP-BEZ235, a dual PI3K/mTOR inhibitor, prevents PI3K signaling and inhibits the growth of cancer cells with activating PI3K mutations. Cancer Res. 2008;68(19):8022–30.
54. Li R, Pourpak A, Morris SW. Inhibition of the insulin-like growth factor-1 receptor (IGF1R) tyrosine kinase as a novel cancer therapy approach. J Med Chem. 2009;52(16):4981–5004.
55. Papaetis GS, Syrigos KN. Sunitinib: a multitargeted receptor tyrosine kinase inhibitor in the era of molecular cancer therapies. BioDrugs. 2009;23(6):377–89.

56. Pietras K, Hanahan D. A multitargeted, metronomic, and maximum-tolerated dose "chemo-switch" regimen is antiangiogenic, producing objective responses and survival benefit in a mouse model of cancer. J Clin Oncol. 2005;23(5):939–52.
57. Ito T, Okusaka T, Nishida T, Yamao K, Igarashi H, Morizane C, et al. Phase II study of sunitinib in Japanese patients with unresectable or metastatic, well-differentiated pancreatic neuroendocrine tumor. Invest New Drugs. 2012;31(5):1265–74.
58. Kulke MH, Lenz HJ, Meropol NJ, Posey J, Ryan DP, Picus J, et al. Activity of sunitinib in patients with advanced neuroendocrine tumors. J Clin Oncol. 2008;26(20):3403–10.
59. Strosberg JR, Weber JM, Choi J, Campos TL, Valone TL, Han G, et al. A phase II clinical trial of sunitinib following hepatic transarterial embolization for metastatic neuroendocrine tumors. Ann Oncol. 2012;23(9):2335–41.
60. Raymond E, Dahan L, Raoul JL, Bang YJ, Borbath I, Lombard-Bohas C, et al. Sunitinib malate for the treatment of pancreatic neuroendocrine tumors. N Engl J Med. 2011; 364(6):501–13.
61. Oberstein PE, Saif MW. Update on novel therapies for pancreatic neuroendocrine tumors. JOP. 2012;13(4):372–5.
62. Ferrara N. Role of vascular endothelial growth factor in physiologic and pathologic angiogenesis: therapeutic implications. Semin Oncol. 2002;29(6 Suppl 16):10–4.
63. Rouhi P, Lee SL, Cao Z, Hedlund EM, Jensen LD, Cao Y. Pathological angiogenesis facilitates tumor cell dissemination and metastasis. Cell Cycle. 2010;9(5):913–7.
64. Folkman J. Tumor angiogenesis: therapeutic implications. N Engl J Med. 1971;285(21): 1182–6.
65. Pavel ME, Hassler G, Baum U, Hahn EG, Lohmann T, Schuppan D. Circulating levels of angiogenic cytokines can predict tumour progression and prognosis in neuroendocrine carcinomas. Clin Endocrinol (Oxf). 2005;62(4):434–43.
66. Kazazi-Hyseni F, Beijnen JH, Schellens JH. Bevacizumab. Oncologist. 2010;15(8):819–25.
67. Yao JC, Phan A, Hoff PM, Chen HX, Charnsangavej C, Yeung SC, et al. Targeting vascular endothelial growth factor in advanced carcinoid tumor: a random assignment phase II study of depot octreotide with bevacizumab and pegylated interferon alpha-2b. J Clin Oncol. 2008;26(8):1316–23.
68. Chan JA, Stuart K, Earle CC, Clark JW, Bhargava P, Miksad R, et al. Prospective study of bevacizumab plus temozolomide in patients with advanced neuroendocrine tumors. J Clin Oncol. 2012;30(24):2963–8.
69. Kulke MH, Siu LL, Tepper JE, Fisher G, Jaffe D, Haller DG, et al. Future directions in the treatment of neuroendocrine tumors: consensus report of the National Cancer Institute Neuroendocrine Tumor clinical trials planning meeting. J Clin Oncol. 2011;29(7):934–43.
70. Chaves J, Saif MW. IGF system in cancer: from bench to clinic. Anticancer Drugs. 2011;22(3):206–12.
71. Furukawa M, Raffeld M, Mateo C, Sakamoto A, Moody TW, Ito T, et al. Increased expression of insulin-like growth factor I and/or its receptor in gastrinomas is associated with low curability, increased growth, and development of metastases. Clin Cancer Res. 2005;11(9):3233–42.
72. Atzori F, Tabernero J, Cervantes A, Prudkin L, Andreu J, Rodríguez-Braun E, et al. A phase I pharmacokinetic and pharmacodynamic study of dalotuzumab (MK-0646), an anti-insulin-like growth factor-1 receptor monoclonal antibody, in patients with advanced solid tumors. Clin Cancer Res. 2011;17(19):6304–12.
73. Reidy-Lagunes DL, Vakiani E, Segal MF, Hollywood EM, Tang LH, Solit DB, et al. A phase 2 study of the insulin-like growth factor-1 receptor inhibitor MK-0646 in patients with metastatic, well-differentiated neuroendocrine tumors. Cancer. 2012;118(19):4795–800.
74. Höpfner M, Baradari V, Huether A, Schöfl C, Scherübl H. The insulin-like growth factor receptor 1 is a promising target for novel treatment approaches in neuroendocrine gastrointestinal tumours. Endocr Relat Cancer. 2006;13(1):135–49.

75. Tolcher AW, Sarantopoulos J, Patnaik A, Papadopoulos K, Lin CC, Rodon J, et al. Phase I, pharmacokinetic, and pharmacodynamic study of AMG 479, a fully human monoclonal antibody to insulin-like growth factor receptor 1. J Clin Oncol. 2009;27(34):5800–7.
76. Srirajaskanthan R, Toumpanakis C, Meyer T, Caplin ME. Review article: future therapies for management of metastatic gastroenteropancreatic neuroendocrine tumours. Aliment Pharmacol Ther. 2009;29(11):1143–54.
77. Schott M, Feldkamp J, Lettmann M, Simon D, Scherbaum WA, Seissler J. Dendritic cell immunotherapy in a neuroendocrine pancreas carcinoma. Clin Endocrinol (Oxf). 2001; 55(2):271–7.

Index

A

AKT pathway
  anticancer activity, 151
  ATP-competitive inhibitors, 152
  cellular proliferation, growth, and metabolism, 147
  everolimus, 146–147, 149–150
  HSP90 inhibitor IPI-504, 151
  IGF/IGFR inhibitors, 156–157
  incidence, 148
  MEN1 gene mutations, 149
  perifosine, 152
  PIP3, 147–148
  PKC inhibitors, 152–153
  pNET tumorigenesis and progression, 146–147
  TSC2 and PTEN, 149
  VEGF synthesis and secretion, 151–152, 155–156
American Joint Committee on Cancer Staging, 84, 85
Array-based comparative genomic hybridization (aCGH), 23
211At-meta-astatobenzylguanidine (MABG), 129
Atrophic gastritis, 36, 46, 90, 118. *See also* Chronic atrophic gastritis (CAG)

B

Bronchial carcinoids, 73

C

Carcinoid tumors
  bronchial carcinoids, 73
  ECL cells, 73
  gastric carcinoids (*see* Gastric carcinoid tumors)
  5-HTP decarboxylase, 74
  loss of heterozygosity, 73
  thymic carcinoids, 72–74
  WDHA syndrome, 74
Chromogranin-A (CgA), 36–37
Chronic atrophic gastritis (CAG), 84, 87, 89
Circulating tumor cells (CTCs), 37–38
CpG island methylator phenotype (CIMP), 23–24

D

Dosimetry, 141–142
Duodenal neuroendocrine tumors, 111, 114–115

E

Endoscopic mucosal resection (EMR), 91
Endoscopic ultrasound (EUS)
  brachytherapy, 111
  CEH–EUS, 105
  curative/palliative management, 111
  diagnostic accuracy, 97–98
  duodenal neuroendocrine tumors, 114–115
  elastography, 105
  EUS–FNA
    core needle/Tru-Cut needle biopsy, 99–101
    cystic PNETs, 96–97, 99–100
    identify pancreatic lesions, 96
    insulinomas size, 96
    tissue acquisition, 98
  functional and nonfunctional symptoms, 95
  gastric carcinoid tumors, 114

J.R. Pisegna (ed.), *Management of Pancreatic Neuroendocrine Tumors*,
DOI 10.1007/978-1-4939-1798-3

Endoscopic ultrasound (EUS) (*cont.*)
gastrinomas, 112
insulinomas
alcohol ablation, 113
radiofrequency ablation, 112–113
intraoperative localization, 104–105
MEN Type 1 patients, 102, 103
nonoperative management, small NF-PNET, 102
photodynamic therapy, 111
preoperative assessment, 104
somatostatinomas, 113–114
Enteropancreatic tumors. *See* Neuroendocrine enteropancreatic tumors (NETs)
Esophagogastroduodenoscopy (EGD), 43
EUS-guided fine-needle aspiration (EUS–FNA)
core needle/Tru-Cut needle biopsy, 99–101
cystic PNETs, 96–97, 99–100
identify pancreatic lesions, 96
insulinomas size, 96
tissue acquisition, 98
Everolimus, 149–150, 153

G
Gastric carcinoid tumors
clinical trial, 93
epidemiology, 84, 85
intramuscular treatments, 92
type I
CAG, 84, 86
clinical presentation, 87
diagnosis, 89–90
mechanism, 87–89
treatment, 91–92
type II
clinical presentation, 87
diagnosis, 89–90
mechanism, 87–89
MEN1/ZES, 86
treatment, 91–92
type III
clinical presentation, 87
diagnosis, 89–90
histologic pattern, 87
mechanism, 87–89
treatment, 92
Gastrinoma
EUS, 112
MEN1, 12
NETs, 69
surgical resection, 122–123
Gastroenteropancreatic-neuroendocrine tumor (GEP-NET), 127
Gastroesophageal reflux disease (GERD), 42
Glucagonoma, 70, 123–124

H
Hypergastrinemia
appropriate hypergastrinemia, 45–46
inappropriate hypergastrinemia, 46–47, 53
MEN1/ZES, 88
spurious hypergastrinemia, 46, 49

I
131I-Metaiodobenzylguanidine (MIBG)
adult dose, 128
albutamol, 128
calcium channel blockers, 128
competitive inhibitor, 128
MABG, 129
norepinephrine analog, 128
phenylephrine and ephedrine, 128
response rates, 128–129
Immunotherapy, 157
11Indium-diethylenetriaminepentaacetic acid (DTPA)-octreotide, 129–130
Inherited syndromes
MEN1 (*see* Multiple endocrine neoplasia type 1 (MEN1))
NF1 gene, 11, 17–18
TSC, 11, 18
von Hippel–Lindau disease
meta-analysis, 15
mutations, 16
protein, 16–17
Insulinoma
EUS
alcohol ablation, 113
radiofrequency ablation, 112–113
laboratory assessment, 35
NETs, 69–70
surgical resection, 121–122

L
Laboratory assessment
clinical features, 34
functioning tumors, 34
non-functioning tumors, 34
non-specific biomarker
chromogranin-A, 36–37
NSE, 37

pancreatic polypeptide, 37
tumor markers, 37
novel biomarkers, 37–38
PTH level, 38–39
serum calcium level, 38–39
specific biomarker
carcinoid syndrome, 35–36
fasting serum gastrin, 34, 35
hypecalcaemia, 35
hypergastrinaemia, 35
insulinoma, 35
Loss of heterozygosity (LOH), 7, 12, 64, 71, 73, 75

M
Mammalian target of rapamycin (mTOR)
anticancer activity, 151
cellular proliferation, growth, and metabolism, 147
everolimus, 146–147, 149–150
HSP90 inhibitor IPI-504, 151
IGF/IGFR inhibitors, 156–157
incidence, 148
patient outcomes, 146
PKC inhibitors, 152–153
pNET tumorigenesis and progression, 146–147
TSC2 and PTEN, 149
VEGF synthesis and secretion, 151–152, 155–156
MEN1. *See* Multiple endocrine neoplasia type 1 (MEN1)
Mixed adenoneuroendocrine carcinoma (MANEC), 3, 5–6
mTOR. *See* Mammalian target of rapamycin (mTOR)
Multiple endocrine neoplasia type 1 (MEN1), 6–7, 11
animal study, 64
classical tumors
NET (*see* Neuroendocrine enteropancreatic tumors (NETs))
parathyroid neoplasia, 65–66
pituitary tumors, 70–71
clinical manifestations, 12, 64–65
definition, 10
gastrinomas and insulinomas, 12
germline mutations, 62–63
inheritance, 64
lactotroph adenomas, 10
menin protein
cell culture, 13
Hedgehog signaling, 15
MLL complex, 14
PRMT5, 15
signaling pathways, 13–14
mutations, 10, 12
nonclassical tumors
adrenal tumors, 74
carcinoid (*see* Carcinoid tumors)
CDKN1B mutations, 76–78
cutaneous manifestations, 75–76
non-pituitary CNS, 71–72
smooth muscle tumors, 75
pituitary adenomas, 10

N
Neuroendocrine enteropancreatic tumors (NETs)
gastrinoma, 69
glucagonoma, 70
insulinoma, 69–70
nonfunctioning, 67–69
octreotide, 66–67
Neurofibromatosis type 1 (NF1), 7, 11, 17–18
Neuron-specific enolase (NSE), 37, 99
Nuclear medicine
PET/CT, 136
PRRT
acute and delayed side effects, 140
administration, 139
dosimetry, 141–142
patient preparation, 139
radiosensitization and chemotherapy, 140
SIRT, 140–141
TACE, 141
somatostatin receptor scintigraphy, 134–135
theranostic approach
contraindications, 138
^{68}Ga and ^{90}Y/^{177} Lu pairs, 136–137
indications, 138
^{111}Indium-octreotide, 137
^{77}Lu-DOTATATE, 137–136
^{90}Y-DOTATOC, 137, 138

P
Pancreatectomy, 118–119, 122
Pancreatic polypeptide (PP), 37, 118
Parathyroid hormone (PTH), 38–39
Parathyroid neoplasia, 65–66
Partial remission (PR), 130

Pathology
  anti-TTF1 antibody, 6
  carcinoid tumor, 5
  familial germline mutations, 6–7
  grading, 3, 5
  incidence, 6
  macroscopic features (T stage), 3–4
  MANEC, 3, 5–6
  nomenclature, 1–2
  SSTR2 receptor, 6
  TNM classification, 2–4
  WHO classification, 2
Peptide receptor radionuclide therapy (PRRT)
  GRPR, 132
  ^{111}In-DTPA-octreotide, 129–130
  locoregional administration, 132
  ^{177}Lu-DOTATOC/^{177}Lu-DOTATATE, 130–131
  nuclear medicine
    acute and delayed side effects, 140
    administration, 139
    dosimetry, 141–142
    patient preparation, 139
    radiosensitization and chemotherapy, 140
    SIRT, 140–141
    TACE, 141
  radiosensitizers, 131
  toxicity, 131
  90Y-DOTATOC, 130
Phosphoinositide 3-kinase (PI3K)
  anticancer activity, 151
  cellular proliferation, growth, and metabolism, 147
  everolimus, 146–147, 149–150
  HSP90 inhibitor IPI-504, 151
  IGF/IGFR inhibitors, 156–157
  IGF-1R receptor, 148
  incidence, 148
  patient outcomes, 146
  PIP3, 147
  PKC inhibitors, 152–153
  pNET tumorigenesis and progression, 146–147
  TSC2 and PTEN, 149
  VEGF synthesis and secretion, 151–152, 155–156
Primary hyperparathyroidism (PHPT), 64–66
Proton-pump inhibitor (PPI) therapy, 42, 45–44
PRRT. *See* Peptide receptor radionuclide therapy (PRRT)
PTH. *See* Parathyroid hormone (PTH)

R
Radiofrequency ablation (RFA), 112–113, 121
RASSF1A, 23

S
Selective internal radiation therapy (SIRT), 140–141
Small intestinal NETs (SINETs), 24
Smooth muscle tumors, 75
Somatic syndromes
  aCGH, 23
  ATRX and DAXX, 20–22
  β-catenin, 18
  epigenetics, 23–24
  expression profiling, 22
  MEN1 (*see* Multiple endocrine neoplasia type 1 (MEN1))
  SINETs, 24
  TSC2 and PTEN, 19
  whole-exome sequencing, 19
Somatostatin receptor subtype 2 (SSTR2), 6, 135, 136
Sunitinib, 153–154
Surgical resection
  functional PNETs
    glucagonoma, 123–124
    somatostatinoma, 124
    VIPoma, 123
  gastrinoma, 122–123
  insulinomas, 121–122
  nonfunctional PNETs
    with liver metastases, 120–121
    localized disease, 118–120
    preoperative assessment and imaging, 118
  postoperative complications, 124

T
Transcatheter arterial chemoembolization (TACE), 121, 141
Tuberous sclerosis complex (TSC), 10, 11, 18

V
Vascular endothelial growth factor (VEGF), 148–149, 155–156
Vasoactive intestinal polypeptidomas (VIPomas), 34, 70
von Hippel–Lindau disease (VHL), 11
  EUS, 96
  germline mutations, 6–7
  meta-analysis, 15

mutations, 16
PI3K/Akt/mTOR pathway, 147
protein, 16–17

W

Whole-exome sequencing (WES), 19, 20, 22

Z

Zollinger–Ellison syndrome (ZES), 12
clinical entity, 42
clinical presentation
diarrhea, 43, 44
EGD, 43
GERD, 42, 44
patient history, 43, 44
PUD, 42–44
radiographic signs, 43, 44
widespread PPI, 44, 45
diagnosis
algorithm, 47–49
hypergastrinemia, 45–47
tumor localization, 50–51
tumor marker, 49
gastric acid hypersecretion, 51–52
medical management, 55–56
surgical management
curative resection, 53
duodenotomy, 52–53
extrapolation, 54–55
long-term survival, 52
MEN-1 patients, 53–54
triangle of Stabile, 52

MIX
Papier aus verantwortungsvollen Quellen
Paper from responsible sources
FSC® C105338

If you have any concerns about our products,
you can contact us on
ProductSafety@springernature.com

In case Publisher is established outside the EU,
the EU authorized representative is:
Springer Nature Customer Service Center GmbH
Europaplatz 3, 69115 Heidelberg, Germany

Printed by Libri Plureos GmbH
in Hamburg, Germany